AROMATICS

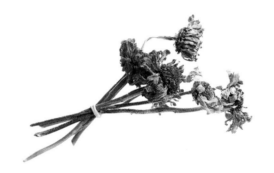

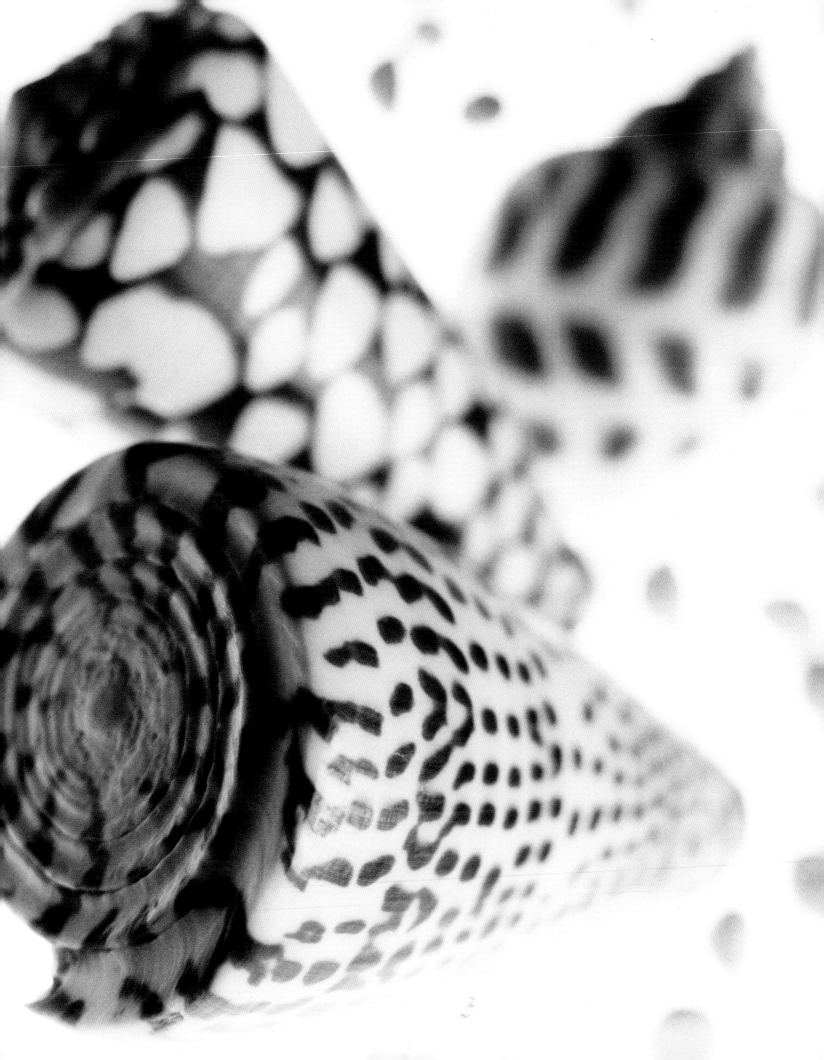

AROMATICS

Angela Flanders

Photography by Simon Wheeler

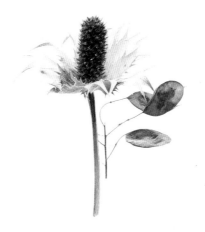

CLARKSON N. POTTER, INC.

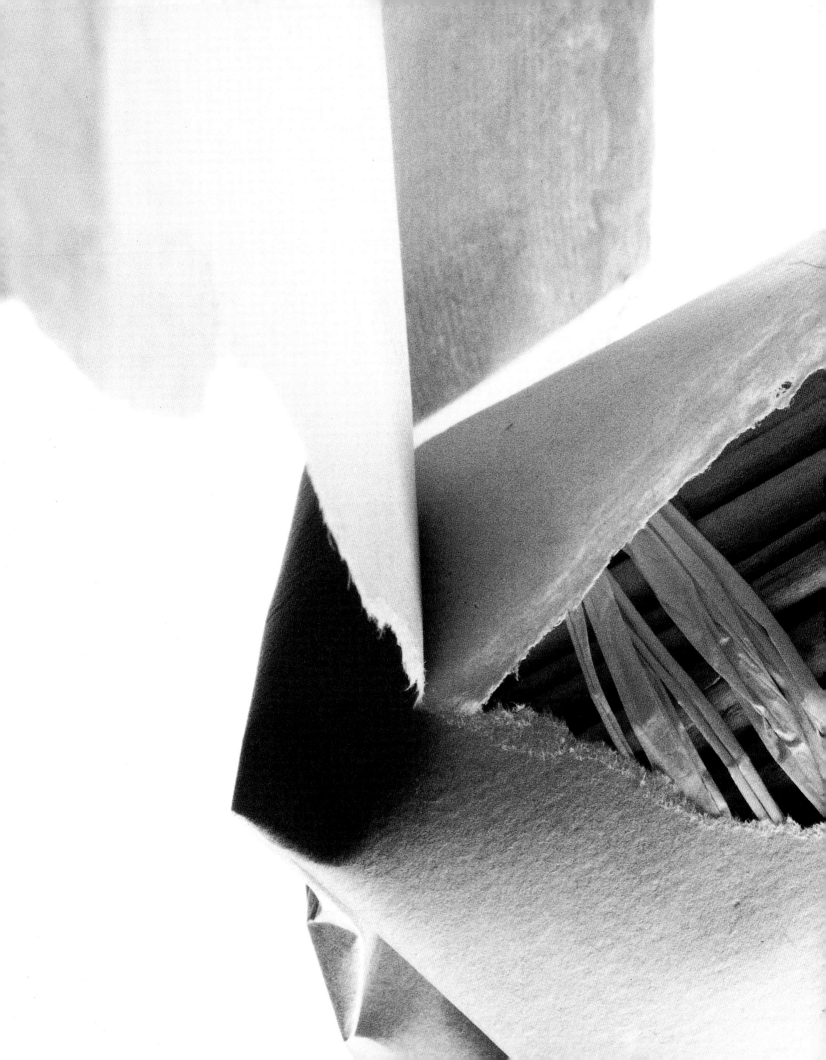

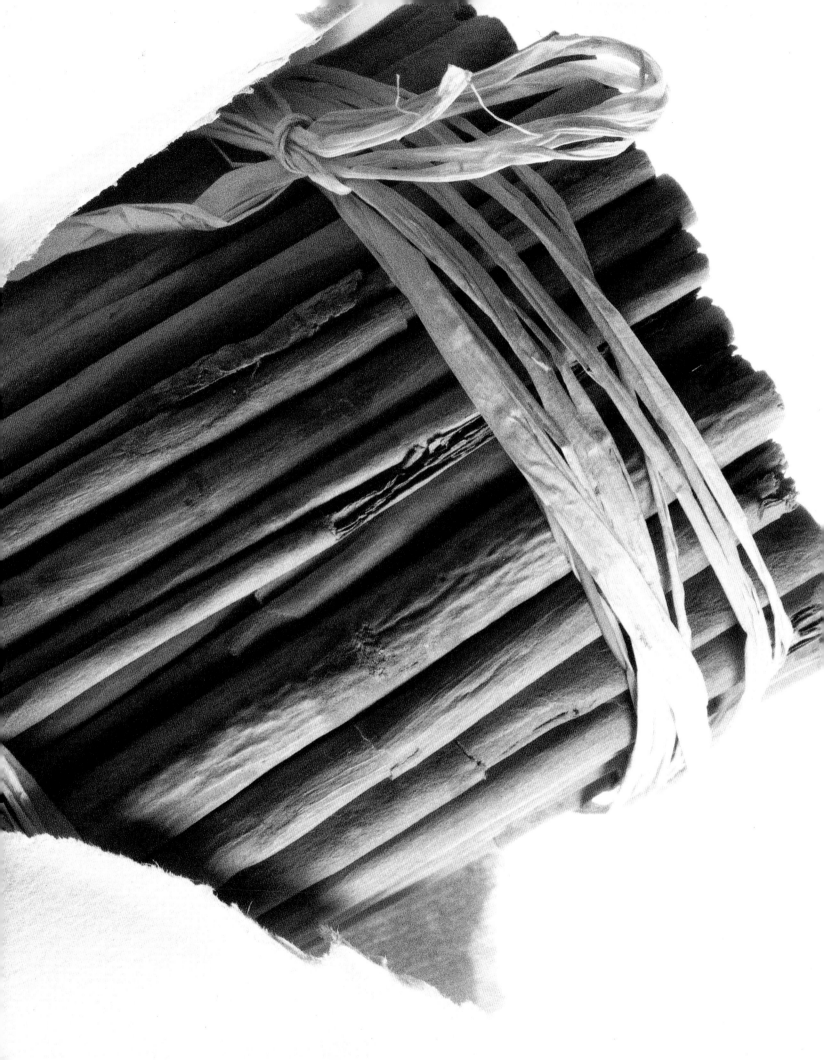

This book is dedicated to my daughter Kate,
with all my love.
And to the memory of Ken, who was so richly
endowed with the priceless gifts of
imagination, humour and courage.
(30.1.56 – 14.5.93)

Text copyright © 1995 by Angela Flanders
Photographs copyright © 1995 by Simon Wheeler

Published by Clarkson N. Potter, Inc., 201 East
50th Street, New York, New York 10022.
Member of the Crown Publishing Group.

Random House, Inc. New York, Toronto,
London, Sydney, Auckland

First published in the United Kingdom in 1995
by Mitchell Beazley, an imprint of Reed
Consumer Books, Michelin House, 81 Fulham
Road, London SW3 6RB and Auckland,
Melbourne, Singapore, and Toronto.

CLARKSON POTTER, POTTER, and colophon
are trademarks of Clarkson N. Potter, Inc.

Manufactured in China

Library of Congress Cataloging-in-Publication
data is available upon request.

ISBN 0-517-70194-4

10 9 8 7 6 5 4 3 2 1

First American Edition

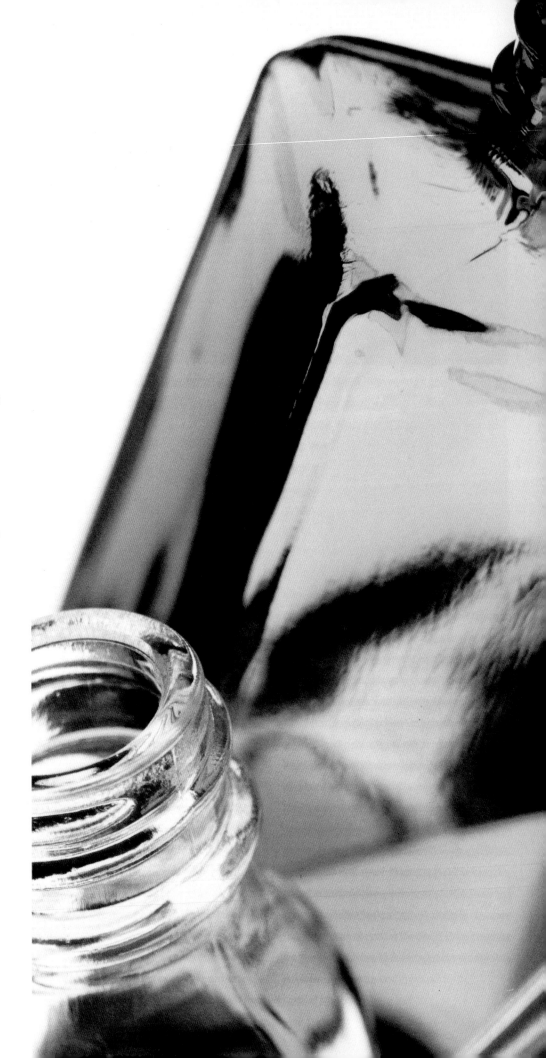

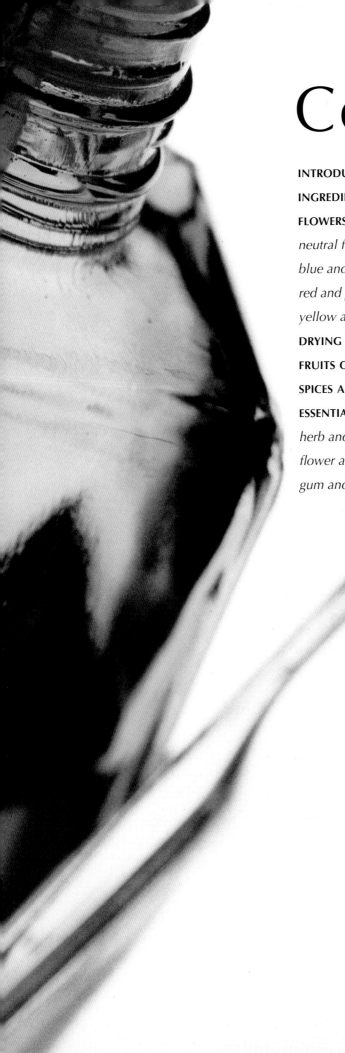

Contents

INTRODUCTION

There is a Chinese proverb which says that the journey of a thousand miles begins with one small step. I wonder how many people have embarked upon that journey without even knowing it, and are well along the road before they even realize that they are traveling! With hindsight, this is what happened to me when, in the spring of 1985, I took on the lease of a small shop in Columbia Road. This historic part of East London is not far from Spitalfields, where the Huguenot weavers settled in England over 300 years ago and produced beautiful silks. The Huguenots loved flowers and singing birds and Columbia Road is said to be a remnant of the many thriving street markets which once abounded in the area; today's flower market has taken place every Sunday morning for over a hundred years.

When I first came to Columbia Road I had no intention of working with flowers, for at that time I was a decorative painter, heavily involved with the magic of paint and faux finishes and painting and restoring antique furniture. Columbia Road is one of the few remaining unspoilt streets of 19th-century shops in London and I soon purchased the next-door shop as well. It had been shut up for 25 years but, hidden behind pegboard and 1940's wallpaper, was a perfect 19th-century shop with all its original features. And so my journey began; I opened the shop intending to sell small antique and decorative furnishings to the many people who came to buy flowers and plants at the market on Sundays. To decorate the shop I dried some flowers and to make it smell good I used some traditional, handmade pot-pourri. The flowers and fragrances took off in a remarkable way and soon I gave up painting to concentrate on the flowers.

I became fascinated by pot-pourris and their fragrances; the ones I sold smelt lovely but my customers were beginning to ask for something different and I realized that the fashion was changing; I pleaded with my supplier for more inventive pot-pourris, but to no avail. Memory took me back to my childhood and to Pendennis, the large house in Derbyshire where I grew up.

To this day I can still recall the slightly musty, floral, spicy and orissy smell of great bowlfuls of pot-pourri that scented the entrance hall of the house. Of all the senses, the olfactory has the greatest ability to awaken memory and a whiff of perfume can take us back years; in the words of the philosopher Jean Jacques Rousseau, "smell is the sense of the imagination."

The pot-pourri making at Pendennis was presided over by Aunt Beth, who wasn't my aunt but was affectionately called so. She made pot-pourris in season, moth herbs, sachets and ointments. I used to follow her around the garden as a small child and she taught me much of what I know of nature. With this background I saw no difficulty in making my own pot-pourri. I remembered a spice mill in East London and called in to buy cinnamon, cloves, cassia and coriander, allspice and nutmeg, orange and lemon peels. I made a trip to Baldwin's wonderful herb shop in the Elephant and Castle to purchase essential oils of orange, cinnamon, bergamot and clove and fixatives of orris root and gum benzoin and much else I couldn't resist. And so my pot-pourri making began. I saturated the small seeds and powders with fragrant oils and left the mix to mature in a large glass jar and forgot all about it. On a busy Sunday before Christmas I suddenly remembered the mix and emptied it into a large bowl and carried it into the shop. The reaction was extraordinary! One man who had made his purchases wanted to know what it was; my Flanders No 1 sold out within the hour and the mix, now called Seville, is still a year-round favorite.

Years on, after countless visits to Baldwin's shop I now have several flower merchants, still the same spice mill, a wonderful gums merchant and two marvelous fragrance men, father and son, who supply me with essential oils. I have been extremely fortunate on my journey, for many people have fed me with knowledge as well as supplies. I now spend most of my time living and working in Dorset, but I will always remember my years in Bethnal Green with great affection.

CHOOSING THE RIGHT INGREDIENTS

Man first discovered perfume by burning fragrant woods, some of which may have contained gum resins. The word perfume comes from the Latin "*pro fuma*" meaning "through smoke," which suggests that the first perfumes were primitive forms of incense. For thousands of years all manner of aromatics have been burnt to release their fragrance, from the scented pastilles of the Middle Ages to the practice of burning scented paper and scent-diffusing lamps in the 18th and 19th centuries. Today you can bring a host of wonderful natural smells into your home simply by using a fragrant oil burner.

The Ancient Egyptians, Greeks and Romans all made lavish use of aromatic substances and the pot-pourris and other fragrant products that we now use to scent our homes are descended from age-old mixes of dried scented flowers, leaves, herbs and spices that have been in existence for centuries.

Modern transport and communications have dramatically lowered the prices of what were once highly prized plant materials and it is hard to imagine that spices that are now so inexpensive and readily available were once so sought-after that men risked their lives to smuggle a few seeds from one country to another. Monopolies were created, wars fought and continents discovered in the search for all kinds of miraculous aromatics: for spices were most valued for their fragrances and they were, and still are, an important part of perfumery.

This book is divided into three broad sections. First comes the Ingredients section which you should study before you try to tackle any of the pot-pourri recipes in the second section, or the other scented projects to make at home described in the third section. Because flowers are often the starting point for creating a pot-pourri or a dried flower arrangement, the Ingredients section opens with an overview of attractive dried flowers grouped according to color. Then there is a practical chapter on how to dry and store flowers and foliage, with instructions for various drying methods including air drying, water drying, how to use desiccants (in particular how to achieve stunning results using silica gel), microwaving for speedy results when time is short and how to preserve foliage to perfection using glycerine.

As well as flowers and foliage there are plenty of other plant materials that contribute to pot-pourri making and scented dried flower arranging – these materials I have collectively called fruits of the earth and include decorative fruits, seed-heads, nuts, cones, woods and barks. In addition there are the all-important spices and fixatives. Spices have always played a vital part in the gentle art of household perfuming and pot-pourri making, and they feature widely in the recipes in this book. All spices have fixative qualities, but they are more powerfully aromatic than a true fixative, which does not usually have an intrusive scent of its own, yet displays great tenacity and often acts as a catalyst drawing other scents together. Most spices are too powerful to fulfil this role, and unless they are used with discretion they can often be identified in a blend – but, of course, it is just that spicy, floral fragrance that typifies a good traditional pot-pourri. Spices vary in price but most are fairly inexpensive. Mixed whole spices can be used as a major ingredient in heavy, woody pot-pourris, while smaller amounts of whole, crushed or powdered spices will add a dry note to a pot-pourri with a rich floral or warm vanilla scent. Especially fragrant spices like cardamom can be used to lend a subtle top note to floral and citrus pot-pourris.

Once you have concocted a well-balanced mix of dried flowers, leaves, herbs, spices and fixatives then all that remains is to scent them with a blend of essential oils. Because some natural essential oils, such as neroli and rose, are extremely expensive, more affordable synthetic versions are processed. Synthetic oils fulfil an important role in blending, although they do not possess the same life-enhancing virtues of their natural counterparts. Nevertheless, it is always worth using natural essential oils whenever possible, because their heavenly scents and special qualities contribute to our general health and well-being. Their virtues are well recognized in aromatherapy, but their therapeutic role in aromatic products for the home (a primary function in the past) has been largely forgotten and although there is a reawakening of interest, many people are still unaware of the astonishing virtues of many natural oils.

An enormous quantity of flowers are needed to produce even a tiny amount of essential oil. For instance, 22lb of lavender flowers produce just 10½oz of oil. Essential oils are always measured and sold by weight, since they vary considerably from a very light and fluid to a thick and viscous consistency. It is useful to remember that on average 2.2lb of oil in weight equals 1¾ pints of liquid measure. When you consider the laborious and often complex processes involved in the production of these precious substances, it is amazing that so many of the wood, spice, herb and peel oils are so reasonably priced. Prices of oils fluctuate, but be suspicious of a range of oils offered at a uniform price – they may not be full strength. I have divided the oils chapter into three categories: floral and fruit oils, herb and spice oils and gum and wood oils. There is also advice on how to blend oils. Note that natural oils are powerful therapeutic agents and can produce headaches and even cause nausea in some sensitive individuals. For a list of hazardous essential oils, see page 141.

THE ART OF POT-POURRI MAKING

Although there are all sorts of ready-made pot-pourris on the market, the ingredients in a commercial pot-pourri are often of limited interest. Making your own pot-pourri is straightforward, particularly if you follow the dry method explained on page 56. By making your own pot-pourri you will produce far more exciting results than purchasing a pre-prepared mix, both in visual and olfactory appeal. If you can bear to give any away then wrapped in cellophane it makes a perfect gift.

When I first began making pot-pourri for my shop years ago I wanted to try and reproduce some of the wonderfully fragrant recipes I remembered from my childhood. Traditional pot-pourri making by the moist method explained on page 48 is a lengthy process. It can involve many months of maturation but the results are excellent because plenty of fragrance can be added with no fear of spoiling the appearance of the flowers with heavy concentrations of powders and oils.

However, I resolved to try and find a way of adapting the traditional moist method. My aim was threefold: to speed up the making process, retain the final quality of scent and improve on the finished visual effect. So I devised my own method of blending fragrant natural oils, herbs, spices and fixatives with dried plant material. Knowing that all plant material will absorb fragrance (albeit to varying degrees) I hit upon a way of distributing the fragrance evenly through the mix. Simply to sprinkle oils on to a dry mixture would mean that heavy concentrations landed only on certain pieces of plant material. Equally, if I diluted the oils and saturated or sprayed the mix then the look of the flowers would be ruined. After careful thought I realized that small-scale ingredients such as seedheads, individual seeds, nuts, berries, small leaves and some spices and woods could be separately soaked with fragrance and allowed to thoroughly absorb it before being added to the rest of the pot-pourri. I refer to these ingredients as carrier materials as they literally transport the perfume throughout the entire mix. I then took this notion a step further by also mixing fixative powders and spices with a small quantity of oil to form a crumbly mix of minute perfumed particles to distribute scent through the mix.

I have used this dry method of pot-pourri making to this day. Sometimes I vary the method according to the nature of the ingredients. For instance, I leave out powders when using dark-colored plant materials in order to prevent the end result looking dusty and drab, but seeds or nuts can be rubbed with oil or soaked in an oil blend to carry the scent instead.

There are three main elements involved in the composition of a successful pot-pourri – the name, the perfume and the plant materials and all of these factors should be in harmony. For example, a name like Primavera (see page 60) gives an instant impression of freshness and is appropriately composed of spring flowers and mosses. In contrast, the more exotically named Zanzibar (see page 86) conjures up a rich, woody concoction full of spicy fragrance. All my pot-pourris are inspired by a composite of a careful blend of perfumes, a balanced choice of plant materials and encapsulated in an evocative name.

I believe that all 30 original recipes take pot-pourri making a considerable step forward; here an ancient art is redefined in a contemporary context. Once you have completed a recipe and topped the mix with an appropriate trimming of, say, a few perfect flowerheads, fruits, seedheads or pressed leaves, the end result is akin to a still life. But beyond the esthetic a well-made pot-pourri is, of course, a refreshable source of delicious scent.

In a break with tradition, the photographs that accompany the pot-pourri recipes present a deliberately free interpretation of the relevant lists of ingredients. By bringing into focus just the trimmings that lend the finishing touches to every recipe I hope you will gain a clear idea of the overall look and character of each pot-pourri. Once you have completed the pot-pourri make your own choice of container: roses and garden flowers are best displayed in china or antique bowls; country flowers and herby mixes sit well in pottery dishes; heavier spicy pot-pourris look wonderful in wooden dishes or bowls and a combination of sea shells and moss impress against glass. Avoid putting pot-pourri in a metal container as it may well interfere with the scent.

After some practice you will find that the main joy of making your own pot-pourri is that there is an enormous diversity of plant materials to work with. Do not be afraid to stray from the ingredients specified in the recipes; if an ingredient is not available simply substitute it for something else. Be bold, experiment and explore the wealth of plant material that is to hand.

CREATING OTHER SCENTED DELIGHTS

As well as making your own pot-pourris to enhance your home, a wide range of dried plant materials and natural oils can be combined to make all sorts of scented delights for use in every room of the house. For instance, with a little time and some basic sewing equipment you can create your own lavender bags and scented sachets, or refresh drawers and closets with scented drawer liners. For the bedroom I have suggested a number of fragrant pillow mixes to soothe and help induce sleep. For the bathroom there are recipes for a selection of perfumed bath oils and soaps. Whatever your skin type, or whether you want to relax and unwind at the end of the day or wake up invigorated in the morning, appropriate oil blends are specified. Perhaps you may be tempted to make scented candles, or add a festive touch at Christmas with traditional pomanders. You can make wooden furniture smell divine with scented polish or send a special letter with fragrant ink and paper. All of these projects would make beautiful gifts.

For those extra-special occasions I have created numerous larger-scale projects to mark the year's passing. The flowers in the mossy spring wreath are a celebration of nature's renewal. The scented summer circle is full of blowsy peonies in all their glory that dry to perfection in silica gel; the shell drop is an ideal way to use up a collection of shells accumulated after a beach vacation, and the delicate hydrangea garland is light and pretty, ideal for decorating a doorway or a buffet table for an open-air party. The spicy mulling ring reflects the mellow fruitfulness of fall and for the winter there is a candelabra perfect for marking the four weeks of Advent and a fir cone swag to provide an impressive Christmas centerpiece.

A summary of the tools and equipment you will need to complete the projects is given on pages 132-3. And finally the plant gazetteer provides a quick and useful reference for the plants covered in the book, however familiar or obscure.

Angela Flanders

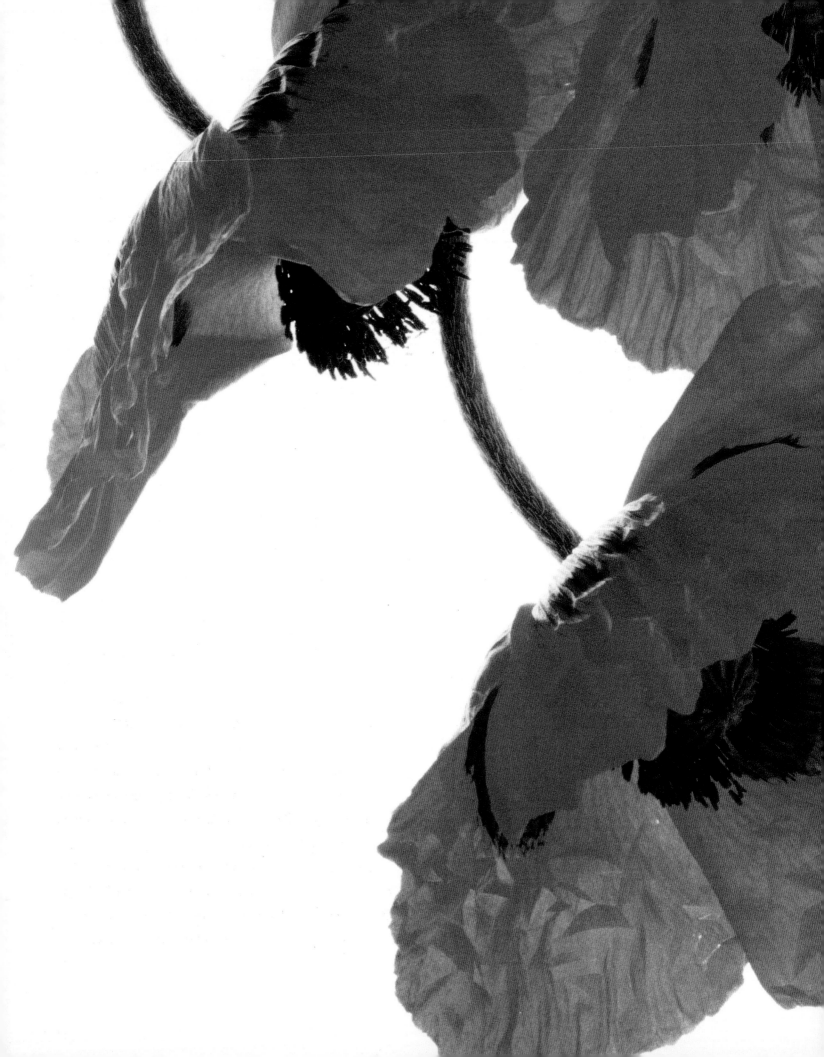

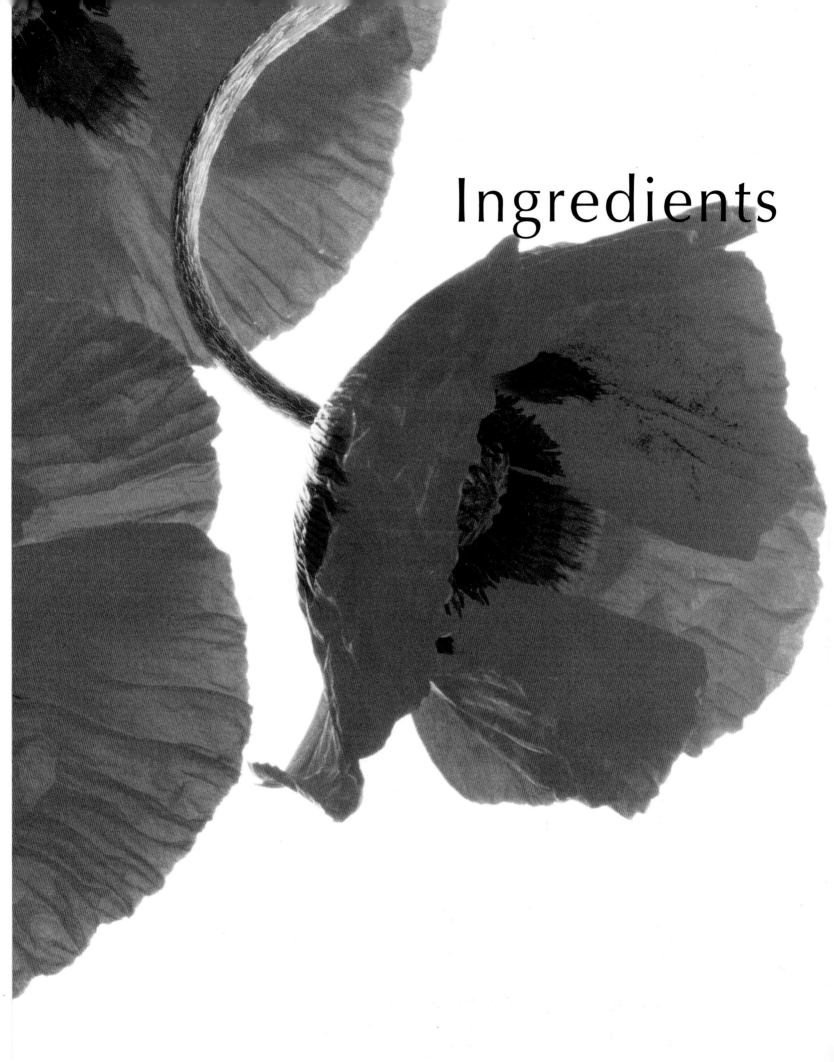

Ingredients

Neutral Flowers

Neutral shades are useful throughout the seasons. Some of those listed are garden plants while others can be found growing wild. White flowers can dry to a drab beige, but the plants listed here retain their clarity of hue well.

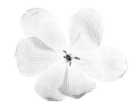

1. HONESTY *Lunaria annua*

You can pick honesty seedpods at an early stage of development when they have a beautiful green and purple coloring and hang them up to air dry. The longer you leave the pods on the plant to ripen, the easier it is to rub off the outer casing to reveal silvery, mother-of-pearl-like "pennies" which are the inner sections of the seedpods.

2. MASTERWORT *Astrantia major*

Starlike masterwort flowers have delicate veined petals. Grow them yourself or buy as cut flowers and hang upside-down in small bunches to dry. Individual heads or small sprays dry well in silica gel. There is also a pink variety which dries to a purplish-pink.

3. EUCALYPTUS *Eucalyptus*

This is the only leaf which retains its gray-green color and its delicious scent when glycerined. It grows all over the world and there are said to be over 200 types ranging from the common round-leaved varieties, through all kinds of oval and pointed types to a fine needle-like leaf. The round-leaved sorts will air dry and retain their color well, while others can turn a lovely purplish-brown when glycerined. Individual dried leaves are endlessly useful in pot-pourris and they mix beautifully with oak moss.

4. ERYNGIUM *Eryngium giganteum*

This particular variety of eryngium is known as 'Miss Willmott's Ghost.' It has a lovely architectural quality, both when growing and when it has been dried. The large flowers have a greenish-purple tinge and the leaves are quite beautiful. Individual heads are ideal for trimming pot-pourris. Try to reserve a few flowers of this biennial plant to go to seed. To dry, leave the cut stems standing up in a pot.

5. LOVE-IN-A-MIST *Nigella damascena*

The large oval seedpod of this flower is shown here. Beautifully striped, it has the advantage of being both bulky and light. It is best picked and dried while still green; if it is picked too late then the color fades. Hang the stems up to dry in bunches of not more than ten stems and do not strip the leaves. Note that the seedpods lose their green and purple coloring as they age and become a warm, biscuit shade. The flowers also dry well; choose a double variety and dry them in the same way as the seedpods.

6. POLYBODY FERN *Polypodium vulgare*

All kinds of fern are enormously useful for making pot-pourris and floral decorations. As a general rule they should be pressed, as they tend to shrivel if hung up to dry. This doesn't matter so much in pot-pourri, but in wreaths and other decorations it is best to lay ferns between sheets of newspaper and place them under a carpet or rug – preferably where they will not be walked on. Treated like this they will dry in a few days and retain their shape. Break up large ferns into small pieces for use in pot-pourri. Do not pick bracken with active spores as they are carcinogenic; leave it until it has dropped its spores and turned color in the fall – used like this it can look pretty in fall and winter mixes.

7. AMMOBIUM *Ammobium*

For drying, it is vital to pick ammobium as soon as the first few flowers show their yellow middles. Picked later, the middles turn black as they dry, but gathered at the correct time and hung up to air dry they retain their pure white coloring. The flowers have a distinct outline and dry well in sprays.

8. BELLS OF IRELAND *Molucella laevis*

A decorative plant with bell-shaped calyces at regular intervals up its tall flower spikes; it is excellent for air drying and glycerining. Pick when the small white blooms in the center of each bell have flowered and gone over and the bells have matured to a firm, papery texture but are still green. Strip off the leaves and hang the stems singly or in bunches. Or, glycerine in a light mix of two parts water to one part glycerine and leave for no longer than 48 hours. Then remove from the glycerine and hang separately upside-down. Hung like this in full sun, the stems and bells will bleach to a rich cream color.

9. SHOO FLY LANTERN *Nicandra*

The large shiny green and black seedpods hang like small lanterns along the branches of this sizeable, spreading plant. Pick when the pods are fully developed but still show green or black. Remove the leaves and hang up to air dry in a dark place, in order to preserve the color. If left on the plant or hung to dry in a sunny spot they will turn brown or beige which can be also be useful.

10. ACHILLEA *Achillea millefolium*

With its small, round, creamy-white flowers, this variety, 'The Pearl,' is aptly named. Pick when the flowers are fully open and on a dry day as any dampness causes the flowers to turn brown when drying. Bunch several stems together and hang them up to air dry.

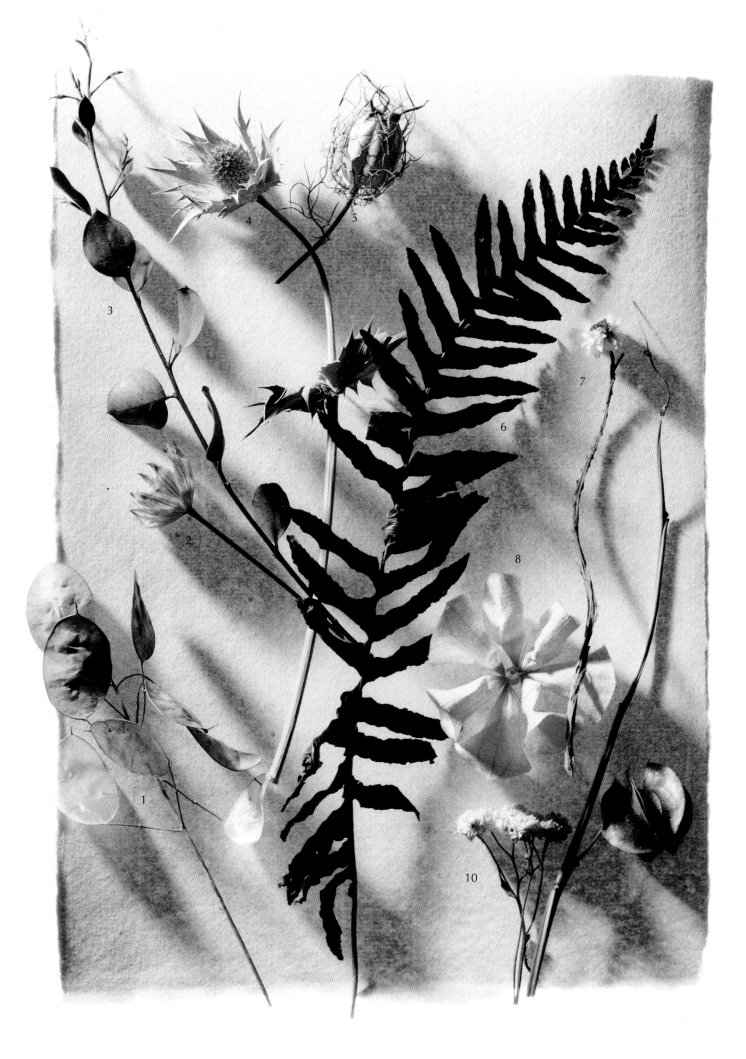

Blue and Purple Flowers

Cool blue, mauve and purple dried flowers keep their colors well over time. Flowers of these hues harmonize with each other, with pinks and reds and contrast well with yellow and orange.

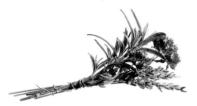

1. DELPHINIUM *Delphinium*

A striking plant which keeps its glorious color well when dried. Delphiniums must be picked at the right time or their petals will drop. Pick when most of the flowers are open but before the bottom flowers start to drop. Hang the spikes upside-down to dry out separately. After a few days, when they feel dry and papery, stand them up to finish drying – this helps them to open up again so they look natural. Use the spikes whole in large arrangements or cut into short sections for wreaths, or as single florets for pot-pourris.

2. HYACINTH *Hyacinthus*

Large, scented spring hyacinths are well worth drying. As they begin to pass their best, snip off the individual florets and dry them in silica gel. Do not attempt to dry the stems as they hold a lot of sap. All shades of hyacinth intensify in color as they dry, in particular the violet-blue kind. Wild hyacinths or bluebells also dry well; they have thinner stems so the whole flower can be dried in silica gel.

3. LAVENDER *Lavandula*

The soft blue spikes of lavender have long been valued for their delicious scent. It derives its name from the Latin "*lavare,*" to wash, and has been used in laundering for centuries. It is an essential part of many pot-pourri recipes, especially the traditional moist ones, where since it has a dry nature it can be used without pre-drying. Pick when the flowers are blue but before they are fully open and hang or stand to air dry.

4. MALLOW *Malva*

This flower is mostly used in pot-pourri mixes. However, perfect specimens of the larger varieties can be glued onto wreaths or swags. The cultivated blue mallow has a rich purplish hue when dried; it is light in weight and texture and so is a useful ingredient in summer and spring mixes. The wild blue mallow is a charming little flower, smaller and lighter in tone than the cultivated type. The large black mallow lends a rich, dark note to exotic pot-pourris. Hollyhock is a type of mallow: the heads dry well air dried (see page 24) or in dessicants (see page 28).

5. HYDRANGEA *Hydrangea*

The color of hydrangeas is affected by the soil in which they grow. Even blue varieties will turn pink in limey soil, whereas in acid soil they will be a beautiful blue. Depending on the variety, they will dry from a pale duck-egg blue, through turquoise to a strong violet blue. Invaluable in summer arrangements and garlands (see pages 124-5), they are also pretty broken into florets in pot-pourris.

6. ERYNGIUM *Eryngium*

The thistle-like heads of eryngium dry very easily. Pick them just before the first tiny flowers come out and hang them up to dry. Do not strip off the leaves which are attractive when dried. Although rather spiky, these flowers make an interesting addition to pot-pourris as a main ingredient or a top dressing. This large 'Zambelii Jewel' variety is most handsome. *Eryngium tripartitum* has small blue oval heads and very blue stems – use this variety in small-scale arrangements.

7. MARJORAM *Origanum*

This plant has long been valued as both a culinary and a medicinal herb. The pinkish-purple flowers, in either the cultivated or the wild varieties, hold their scent well when dried, and both the flowers and the leaves are scented. A good addition to moist and dry method pot-pourris, the sprigs also blend nicely with lavender and other herbs in a dried garland or bunch. Pick when fully out and hang up to dry in a warm, dark place.

8. ACHILLEA *Achillea*

Although similar to marjoram, achillea does not carry any scent. This variety, 'Cerise Queen,' is large and dries to a soft pinkish-mauve which looks delightful mixed with old-fashioned roses and stocks in a floral wreath or garland. Achillea is useful in pot-pourris where the perfume of marjoram is not suitable. Pick when fully out and hang up in bunches to dry in a warm, dark place.

9. AGERATUM *Ageratum*

The small violet-blue flowers of ageratum dry well if they are picked when nearly all the small bobbles are fully out. Wired together in bunches, they are useful in all sorts of dried flower arrangements. The flowers in sprays or as separate blossoms give a striking note in summer or spring pot-pourri.

10. CARDOON *Cynara cardunculus*

Cardoons have spectacular seedheads. They grow up to six feet tall with wonderful silver leaves. Dry after the purple flowers have gone over. Remove the dried brown stamens to reveal the creamy middle surrounded by a shiny silvery calyx. The closely related globe artichoke (*Cynara scolymus*) can be dried at any stage of its growth, from the budlike edible stage through the purple-tufted flowering stage, to the eventual powder-puff seedhead.

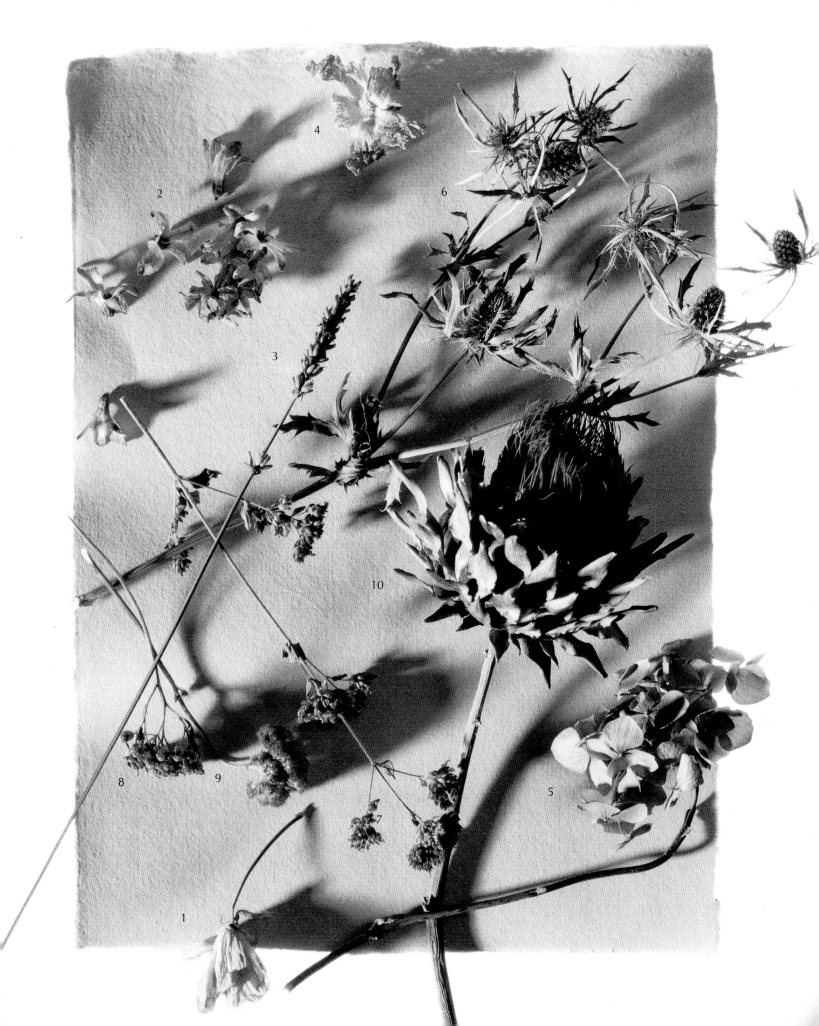

Red and Pink Flowers

Some of the most striking flowers fall into this color category. Pinks and reds are fitting for all seasonal blends in pot-pourris and floral decorations. They are complemented by blues and purples and can be made to look warmer when contrasted with a range of greens.

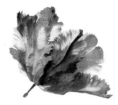

1. COCK'S COMB *Celosia cristata*

When dried, the plushy heads of cockscomb look like crumpled velvet, and they will also absorb and hold fragrance well. Large pieces make a delightful contrast with smooth rose petals in pot-pourris. The velvety texture also gives a seasonal richness to winter mixes and contrasts well with blue pine and all kinds of fir cones. To dry, hang in a warm place.

2. BOUGAINVILLEA *Bougainvillea*

The showy bracts of bougainvillea make a lovely pot-pourri ingredient. These mauve-pink light and fluffy flowers hold fragrance well and blend beautifully with many shades of pink, blue and mauve in a summery mix. Bougainvillea grows in warm climates; if it does not grow locally you may find it available at herb and dried flower suppliers.

3. GLOBE AMARANTH *Gomphrena globosa*

Small globe amaranth flowers are light in weight and absorb fragrance well, so they have long been popular ingredients for pot-pourri making. They range in color from a pale pinkish-white to the rich pink shown here. To dry, cut the stems quite short and hang them up by their stems in small bunches. Once dried, the flowers can be used in small sprays or wired bunches.

4. CARNATION *Dianthus caryophyllus*

These charming flowers have always been valued for their clove-like scent. Some varieties feature in many old still-room recipes and moist pot-pourris. Although modern varieties are larger and the color range far wider, they still lend a traditional touch to floral mixes and decorations. If you air dry them in bunches they shrink and lose their shape, but they, and their gray-green buds, are still useful in pot-pourris. For absolute perfection, dry them in silica gel.

5. STRAW FLOWER *Helichrysum bracteatum*

One of the best-known of all dried flowers, straw flowers come in a broad range of colors, from silver-pink through to dark red. They are very easy to grow and dry. Harvest them while the heads are still closed as they will open as they dry.

6. POLYGONUM *Polygonum bistorta*

The long pink spikes of these flowers can sometimes be found growing wild in water meadows or near rivers. Along with the larger garden variety, *Polygonum bistorta* 'Superbum,' they dry beautifully. With all varieties, pick when fully out and hang upside-down to dry in bunches. Use the long spikes to give strong vertical lines and shape to all kinds of flower arrangements, or else arrange as a top dressing on pot-pourris.

7. PINK PEPPERCORNS *Capsicum*

While most fruits and berries shrivel or drop in the drying process, these last well. They are available from specialist dried flower stores and although quite fragile to handle they hold well once in place. Wired in small bunches or secured with a glue gun, they are a decorative addition to all kinds of dried arrangements. They have no scent of their own, but absorb fragrance well.

8. ROSE *Rosa*

Roses come in every shade of pink and red from the palest shell-like hue to deepest wine. The hundreds of different varieties available today offer an extensive choice of shape and size. The sprays of tiny-flowered rambling roses air dry well. Highly scented old-fashioned shrub roses are valuable in both moist and dry pot-pourris. If you pick perfect specimens of large-flowered hybrid tea roses when they are about half to three-quarters open and hang them up to dry in bunches they will shrink substantially; it is best to dry them in desiccants.

9. PEONY *Paeonia*

The large blooms of peonies are available in pink, red and white. The red is the first to flower and dries well either air dried or as large single heads in desiccants. The huge double pink varieties also dry to frilly perfection in silica gel. Whole flowers or separate petals are pretty ingredients for pot-pourris, but be warned, moths are drawn to peonies and they lay their eggs in the fresh buds. To avoid damage to the flowers, pick peonies for drying when the blooms are half open and, once dry, place in the freezer for 24 hours. This is usually sufficient time to kill any grubs which may be present and prevent them hatching out and damaging the petals.

10. ZINNIA *Zinnia*

These flowers with their fleshy, firm daisy-like heads come in an amazing range of colors from light greenish-pink, through pinks and salmons with a curious fluorescent quality to bright vermilion red. Choose many-petalled double varieties for drying and hang in small bunches to air dry in a cool place, otherwise they tend to shrivel. They also dry very well in desiccants.

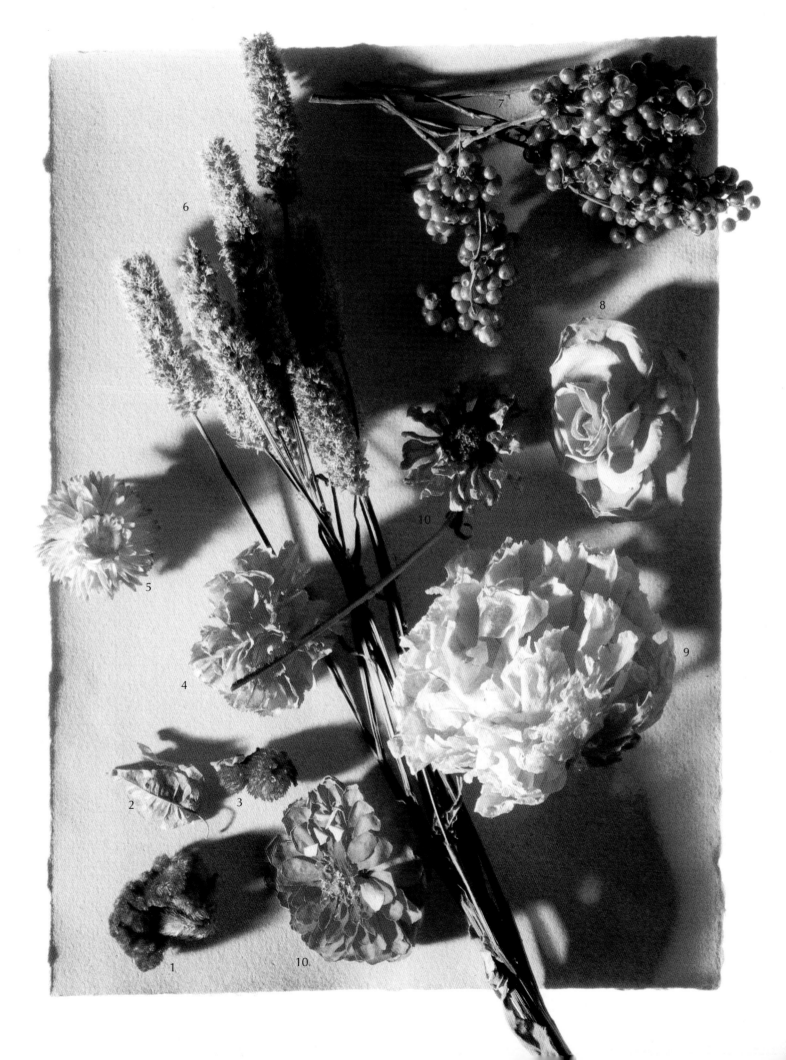

Yellow and Orange Flowers

Although yellow and orange flowers are usually associated with spring and fall, these lively colors give accent and can lift the spirit at any time of the year. They blend well with whites and creams, both are complemented by greens and they make a superb contrast with blue and purple.

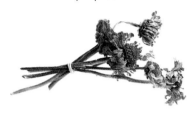

1. AFRICAN MARIGOLD *Tagetes erecta*

These frilly flowers display a huge color range of saffrons, lemons and oranges. The blooms retain their form very well air dried or dried in desiccants. Because of their strong form and rich color they are useful in floral decorations, but use them with care in pot-pourris as they have a very distinct smell which may not blend with the rest of the mix; they are best used in herby and citrus blends.

2. MIMOSA *Mimosa*

A few fresh sprays of delicate, fluffy mimosa will fill a room with fragrance. Alas, cut mimosa does not retain its fluffy quality for long as the flowers shrink as they mature indoors, but do not throw the stems away. They will dry beautifully either hanging in bunches or standing in a small measure of water. The flowers retain their fresh yellow color well and are immensely useful in all kinds of floral decorations and spring pot-pourris as a main ingredient or a top dressing.

3. YARROW *Achillea filipendulina*

There are many different types of yarrow; the striking 'Gold Plate' variety is shown here. Pick this type when the flowers have formed a mass of little bobbles and hang the stems upside-down to air dry. These flowers will dry out quickly almost anywhere, even in quite cool conditions. They are useful for all kinds of dried-flower work and can be broken into sprigs for use in pot-pourris; they are most useful in the lemony, citrus mixes.

4. ROSE *Rosa*

Few dried flowers can compete with the rose as a decorative flower. Yellow roses have a special beauty; some keep their scent well when dried but sadly they do not always retain their color. However, they do turn the most delightful rich creams and tobacco browns when they mature.

5. POLYANTHUS *Primula*

These cheerful little flowers epitomize the spring. They have prolific blooms and some modern hybrids have large flowers in a wide range of golden-yellows, oranges and coral reds. The closely related and much-loved primrose grows wild and has pale yellow blossoms and fresh green leaves; pick these with care as these pretty flowers are not as common as they used to be. Do not air dry *primulas* as they tend to shrink and lose their shape; instead dry them in desiccants for use in pot-pourris and floral decorations.

6. STINKING IRIS *Iris foetidissima*

This memorably named plant grows wild in woods and on chalky ground; it can be very prolific. If you have the right conditions in your garden it is easy to grow and well worth the trouble. In the northern hemisphere the seedheads (shown here) split open in late November to early December to reveal bright orange berries within. These remain smooth and waxy for some time but look equally stunning when they start to shrivel. They become darker in color but are still held in the pea-like pod.

7. TULIP *Tulipa*

This is perhaps not a flower that you would automatically consider drying. Yet all tulips respond well to drying, whether the single tulips, the lily-flowered and frilled-centerd double varieties or the astonishing feather-edged stripy parrot tulips. In every shade of cream to golden-yellows and oranges, splashed and striped together, they will air dry beautifully as single heads when they have fully opened. You can either leave them to dry in a sieve or a basket in a warm place, or, for best results, dry the heads in desiccants so they keep their glorious shapes.

8. CHRYSANTHEMUM *Chrysanthemum*

These familiar flowers are widely available and inexpensive to buy. The small-headed varieties dry well, while the larger ones do not. This 'Primrose Gem' was hung upside-down to air dry. You can also dry the small heads in desiccants.

9. SUNFLOWER *Helianthus annus*

Although sunflowers are rather large to use whole in pot-pourri making they do provide a very useful source of yellow petals for the purpose. While they are suitable for some floral decorations, a miniature type, actually called *Actinella grandiflora*, can be dried whole if smaller heads are required.

10. DAFFODIL *Narcissus*

Perhaps daffodils seem an unlikely choice for drying, but the double varieties in particular will air dry beautifully. Either cut the stems short and hang them to dry upside-down in small bunches, or dry them flat on racks or in baskets. However, of the many kinds of daffodils now available most are best dried in desiccants to preserve their distinctive shapes. Scented narcissi are an important ingredient of traditional pot-pourri recipes.

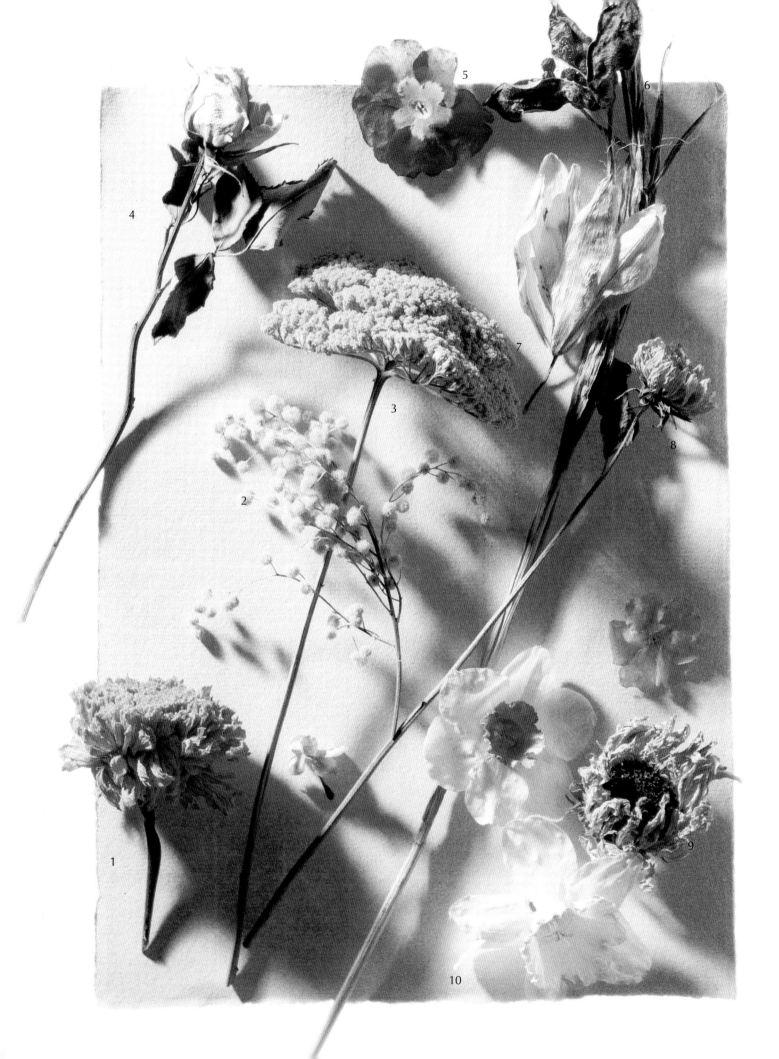

Drying and Storing Flowers

DRYING

There are five main methods of drying and preserving flowers and other plant material for use in pot-pourris and dried flower decorations. These include: air drying (which involves hanging up the flowers or laying them flat), water drying, using desiccants, microwaving, and preserving in glycerine. Whichever method you choose, it is essential that you pick the flowers at the right time and in the right condition.

First, the flowers must be dry. If there is any moisture left on the surface of a flower it will inevitably turn brown during the drying process. Pick flowers from the garden on a dry day after the dew has evaporated, and take particular care when purchasing roses and similar cut flowers, as they may have been sprayed with water to keep them fresh; in this case drying may be unsuccessful.

Secondly, the flowers must be picked at the right stage of development. The color of a flower does not improve once it has been picked, although it may intensify during the drying process. In fact, flowers tend to "blue" as they dry. A fresh, clear pink rose, for example, dries to a mauve-pink and bluish-pinks dry almost to lilac. Also, if you want an apricot or coral-colored dried rose, you should choose light orange or flame-red varieties. A dark red rose will dry almost black. Bear these points in mind when choosing roses, and other flowers for drying.

Some flowers continue to develop as they dry. Larkspurs, for example, will drop their petals if all the flowers on the spike are open when it is hung up to dry. For this reason you should pick larkspur while the flowers at the tips are still in bud, and dry a selection of open flowers, half-open flowers and buds for a natural effect. Some flowers may shrivel if they are picked too soon. Hydrangeas are a good example of this problem so it is vital that these most beautiful and useful flowers are picked at just the right moment. With hydrangeas, what most of us think of as the petals are actually the sepals: the real flowers are the tiny centers, and it is only when these have finished flowering that the sepals begin to change color and thicken. When they develop a thick, leathery texture they are ready to pick and dry, but make sure that you catch them before the first frosts or they can turn brown overnight.

Flowers for drying should not be left lying around once they have been picked. It is important to prepare and begin drying flowers as soon as possible after picking so that they retain their form and color.

STORING

Light and damp are the deadly enemies of all dried plant materials. To protect from both these elements always store dried materials in large cardboard boxes (which will also protect them from dust) in a dark, dry place. Acid-free tissue paper can be layered between more fragile varieties, while glycerined leaves are best stored between sheets of newspaper. Do not pack too much dried plant material into a single box, as the stems may crush each other and so become damaged. However, it is worth noting that squashed or tired-looking dried flowers can often be revived by holding them in the steam from a boiling kettle for a few seconds. If you are storing several boxes of dried plant material it helps to label them.

AIR DRYING (HANGING)

This is the simplest, most commonly employed and usually the best method of drying plant material. Most stems should be hung upside-down, but feathery, light flowers like gypsophila and alchemilla are best dried standing upright in baskets or boxes, with enough space between bunches or single stems for the air to circulate.

1. Strip any untidy leaves off the stems. The fewer leaves there are on the stem the faster the drying process. If the foliage is attractive leave some in place, or else dry the leaves separately (see the flat method of air drying that is explained overleaf.)

2. Make up bunches of not more than ten stems and secure tightly with an elastic band. Large flowerheads or spikes such as delphiniums, artichokes and peonies should be dried separately, or in bunches of two or three.

3. Make a wire S-shaped hook from a short length of 18 swg (see page 132) florist's wire or by opening out a paper clip. Slip one end of the hook under the elastic band and hook the other end on to a line suspended in a dimly lit, warm, dry and well-aired place. Or hang with pegs. Wire coathangers make good supports for small quantities of flowers.

4. When the flowers feel dry, papery and crisp, and the stems are dry and warm to the touch all the way up, the plant material is ready to use or store. The length of drying time depends entirely on the type of plant and the thickness of the stem – some will be ready in a few days, others can take many weeks. Flowers and leaves for use in pot-pourris should have their stalks stripped off at this stage and stored separately. The stems take up a lot of space and will not be needed.

OPPOSITE: *Ranunculus stems are hung upside down and pegged to a line to air dry.*

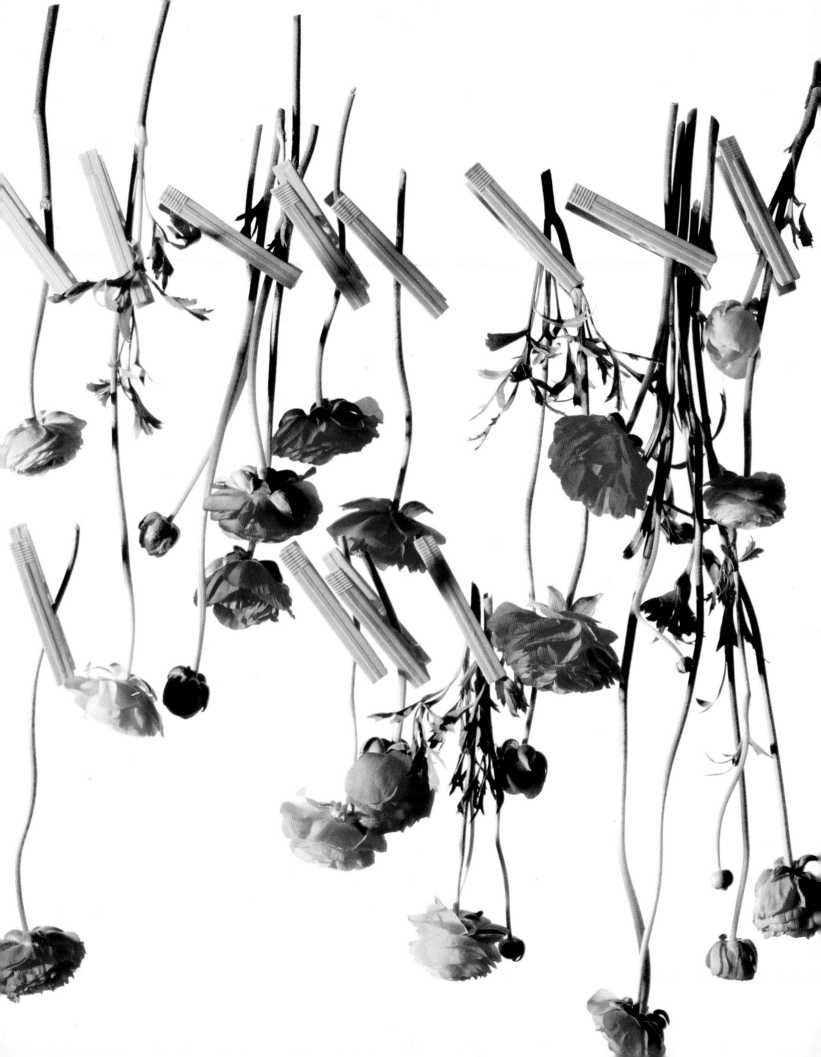

AIR DRYING (FLAT)

This method is ideal for drying loose petals or flowerheads (without stems) for use in pot-pourris; flowerheads can be put to dry even when fully open. The basic requirements of air circulation, warmth and dim light described on the previous page still apply. If you grow or buy a lot of flowers for pot-pourri making, and have enough space, it is worth making up some drying frames from light timber with muslin tacked or stapled to stretch across the frame – then simply lay the flowers and petals on the muslin to dry out naturally. For heavier plant materials you can substitute fine wire mesh for the muslin to provide a more rigid drying frame or, for small quantities of flowers, little shallow baskets, which will look pretty as the flowers are left to dry around the house. Just keep them out of direct sunlight and make sure that the air can circulate around them.

1. To dry petals, spread them out in a single layer on a flat surface where air can circulate and speed the drying process.

2. To dry whole flowerheads in this way, cut the stems as short as possible and lay them face up leaving plenty of space in between.

3. To dry leaves and herbs in this way, spread them out in a single layer, leaving space between them for the air to circulate.

WATER DRYING

This may seem to be a contradiction in terms, but water drying is the best method for drying certain types of flowers. For example, gypsophilia, hydrangea, artemesia and even tulips respond very well to this treatment. Wild flowers like meadowsweet and Queen Anne's Lace also dry well by this method; they retain the natural quality of their stem movement, and are less likely to wilt.

1. Stand the flowers in a vase or container with aproximately ½-1in of water in the bottom of the vessel.

2. Place the container and the flowers in a warm, dimly lit spot.

3. The flowers will slowly drink the water and the drying process will begin. They can be left quite safely until completely dry.

USING DESICCANTS

Different types of desiccants have been used for centuries to draw moisture from the petals of flowers and dry them to an almost perfect state. Sand has long been an agent for drying plant materials, and I traced a recipe from 1609 extolling the virtues of this method. Borax and alum were often used and still are; they are especially useful when mixed with modern, more expensive desiccants as a means of "stretching" them. Silica gel is the most reliable of all modern desiccants and has the advantage of being easy to use.

Sand

This is one of the least costly and oldest drying agents with much to recommend it, although it is time-consuming to prepare. Be certain to obtain fine silver sand which is clean, rather than builder's sand which you will have to wash thoroughly and dry before use. For small quantities, the kind of sand sold in pet stores for use in birdcages is ideal; you can also buy silver sand in large bags. It is sold as dry, but it needs further drying before use. Although some good results can be achieved using this drying agent, sand drying can be a lengthy business. Note that sand can be mixed with borax (three parts sand to one part borax) in order to speed the drying process. Silica gel can be used in the same way; the blue crystals change color to show that the drying is complete.

1. First dry the sand thoroughly. To do this put the sand in shallow metal bowls or baking dishes in a low oven and once dry store in an airtight container in a warm place. The fine sand particles act as a perfect support for every part of the flower.

2. Put a 1in layer of sand in the base of a shallow cardboard box and lay the flowers on top, face up. Gently fill the middle of the upright flowers with sand, using a small spoon. Fill the surrounding space, making sure that the petals are supported by sand and that the flowers keep a good shape, until the blooms are completely covered.

3. If you can place the box in a warm, dry place such as in a boiler space or in an airing cupboard, there is no need to seal it, as any moisture in the sand will be drawn out. Otherwise, seal the box firmly.

4. Leave for up to three weeks before you uncover the flowers. In fact, the flowers can remain in the sand for an unlimited period, as they cannot be overprocessed, unlike with silica.

5. Remove the flowers very gently as they will be fragile and pouring off the sand too quickly may damage them. Trickle the sand off one flower and make sure that it is crispy dry; then the rest of the flowers can be exposed. Use a soft camel hair brush to very gently remove the surplus sand from the surface of the flowers.

6. Store the flowers in airtight containers. A spoonful of silica will help to keep them dry.

Borax

This powder is less expensive than silica, but it tends to leave a white deposit on the flower petals. It does not run down into the petals like sand or silica, and can be mixed with cornmeal in a 50/50 combination. Borax works quite well following the method for silica gel, but it is not as quick or effective.

OPPOSITE: *Beautiful heads of pale tulips are placed on a sieve and left to air dry flat in a warm place.*

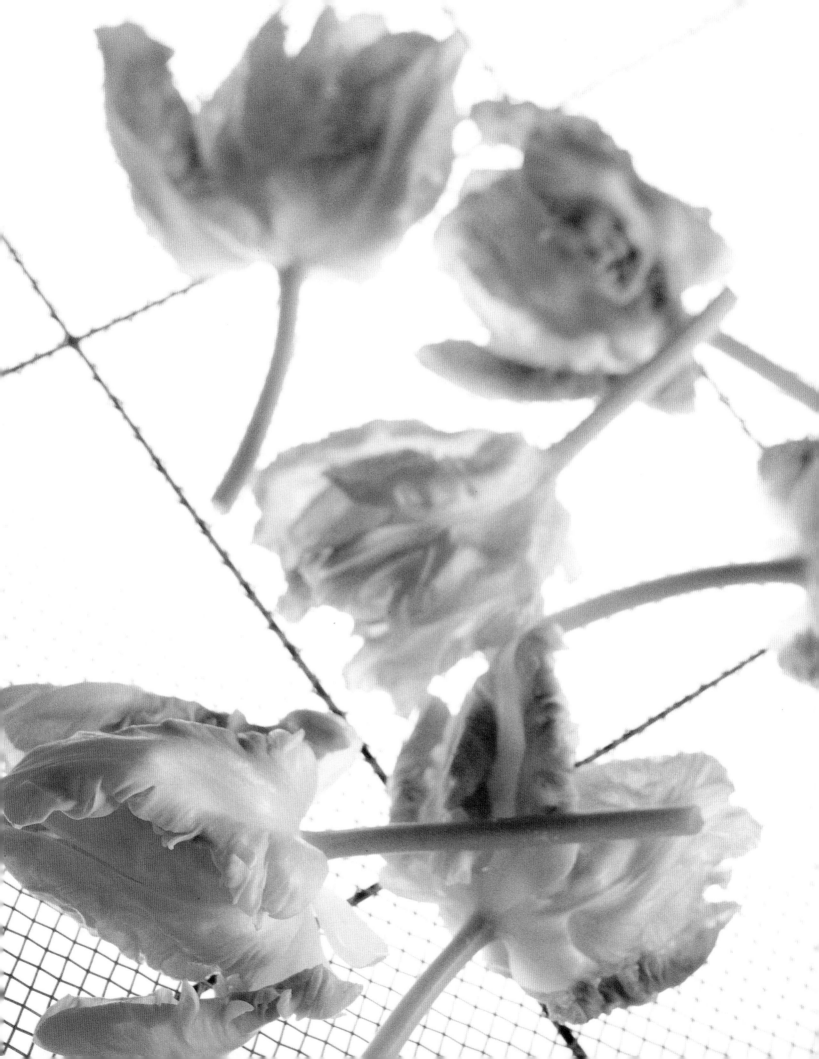

Alum

Another powder used as a drying agent, alum has the same drawbacks as borax and is hard to clean off the dry petals: dust it off with a fine, soft brush. Follow the method for silica gel.

Silica Gel

Although silica gel is quite costly to buy, it is an economical method of drying because it can be used over and over again. It works fast and indicates what it is doing, for it contains some crystals which are brilliant blue when really dry. As the silica draws the moisture out of the petals the crystals turn pink. After use, put the silica in a shallow dish or on a baking tray in a warm oven until the indicating crystals turn blue again; this brings it back to full strength. Store dry in an airtight container. Flowers dry well in silica in a plastic box and dry best in sand in a cardboard box.

1. Cover the base of a suitable container such as a plastic box with a well-fitting lid, to a depth of approximately ½in with dry silica gel. Lay the flowers on top. Most flowers should be placed face up but lay flowers with large, flat heads face down.

2. With a spoon, gently fill the middle of the flowers with silica gel, then fill up the surrounding space; make sure that the petals are supported so the flowers keep a natural shape. Fill the container until the flowers are completely covered. If drying very small, flat flowers you may be able to fit several layers in each container; cover each individual layer of flowers before starting the next.

3. Seal the container. Allow about five days drying time for large flowers like peonies; smaller blooms will take two to three days.

4. When the flowers are dry, gently pour the silica gel off them. Store the dried flowers in airtight containers with a spoonful of dry silica gel in each container.

MICROWAVE DRYING

If you need a few special flowers in a hurry and there is no time to wait for a desiccant to work in the normal way, then the microwave comes into its own. This method is very useful if you have a fine crop of special flowers and a limited quantity of silica, as it speeds up the drying process considerably.

1. Spread a 2in layer of silica gel over a shallow glass or pottery dish. Cut the stalks of the flowers to approximately ½-1in and place them stem down in the silica. Cover the flowerheads gently with more silica, with a spoon, until they are submerged.

2. Place half a cup of water in the microwave with the container and "cook" at full power for two to four minutes, depending on the size of the flowers. Leave the flowers in the silica for some time after this (overnight if possible) and certainly until they are cool.

3. Pour the silica gently off the flowers and dry it for re-use. The flowers can be used at once or stored for future use.

PRESERVING IN GLYCERINE

This is the very best way of preserving both deciduous and evergreen foliage. During the process the water content of the leaves is replaced by glycerine, which leaves them looking totally natural, flexible, supple and sometimes shiny. Inevitably the color changes, and it is impossible to keep the leaves green by this method. However, this is more than compensated for by the amazing range of colors which emerge: everything from palest cream, through every shade of golden-brown and gray, to deepest glossy, brownish-blacks. The leaves retain their final color and form for many years and can be used again and again. They seem only to improve with age and eucalyptus leaves even keep their scent. If the leaves get dusty they can simply be washed in tepid water and gently dried. Choose well-shaped branches with largely undamaged leaves; remove any leaves which are torn or damaged. Pick deciduous foliage once it is mature and while the sap is still rising. When the sap ceases to rise and the fall coloring begins to show a natural seal will form and the stems are then unable to absorb the glycerine. Start to preserve deciduous foliage from mid-summer onward until the leaves begin to turn color. Glycerine evergreen foliage between fall and spring, when it is neither making new growth nor dropping old leaves.

1. Make up a solution of one part glycerine to two parts very hot water. Most plants work well in this, but very heavy leaves can take an equal solution of glycerine and water.

2. Prepare the bases of the stems by splitting the ends with a sharp knife, or else by means of a few hammer blows; they will then take up liquid much more readily. Place them in a narrow, heavy container, with about 4in of glycerine solution in the bottom. Place the container in a dimly lit position for at least a week, although with some types of foliage the process can go on for many weeks. Watch the leaves to monitor the drying: they should remain supple, and when ready the veins will be more distinct and the color will have begun to change.

3. Bunch the stems and hang them upside-down for a week or more (depending on the leaves). By reversing them the solution continues to flow down into the leaf system.

4. If droplets should appear on the leaves, this means have become saturated with the solution and should be taken out of the mixture and washed in warm water, then dried and stored for future use.

OPPOSITE: *A sprig of beech leaves dries to best effect left standing in a jar of glycerine.*

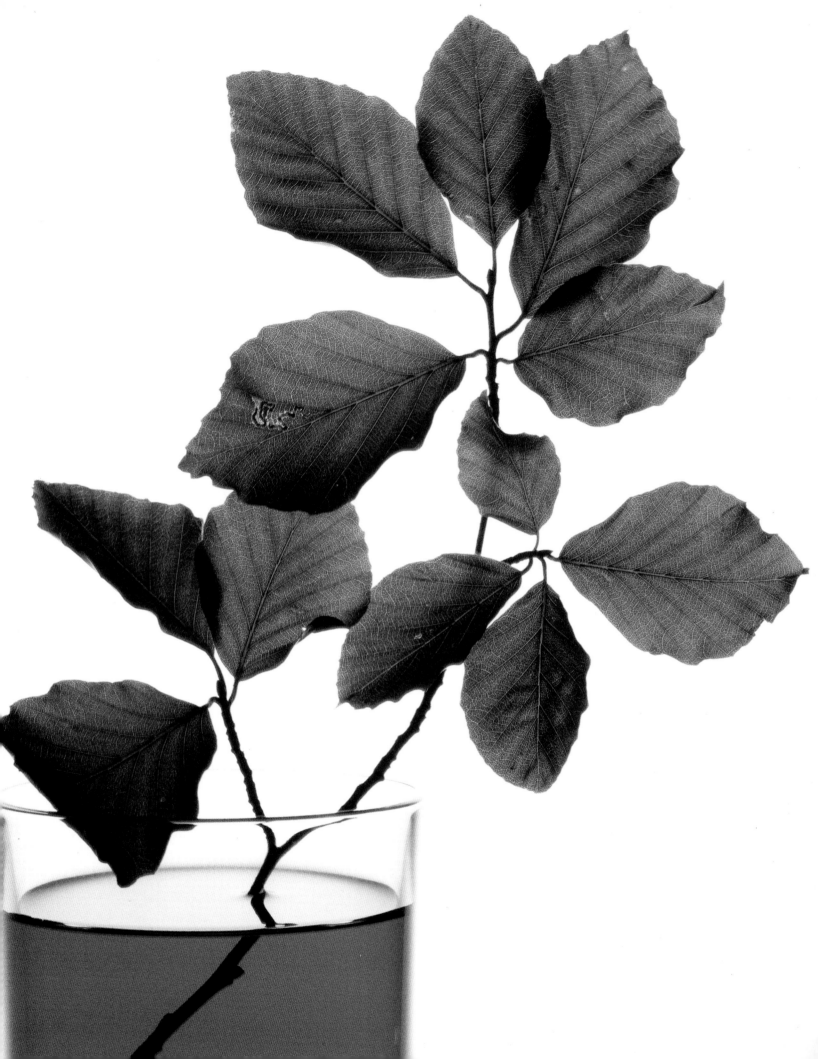

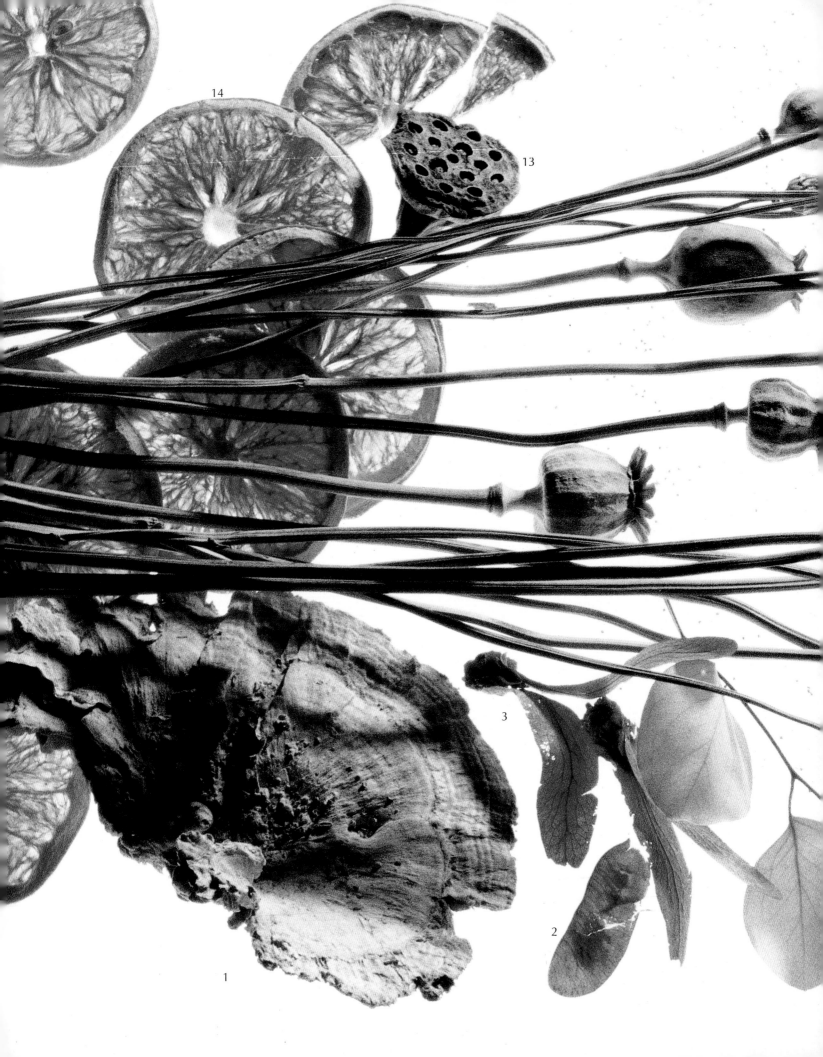

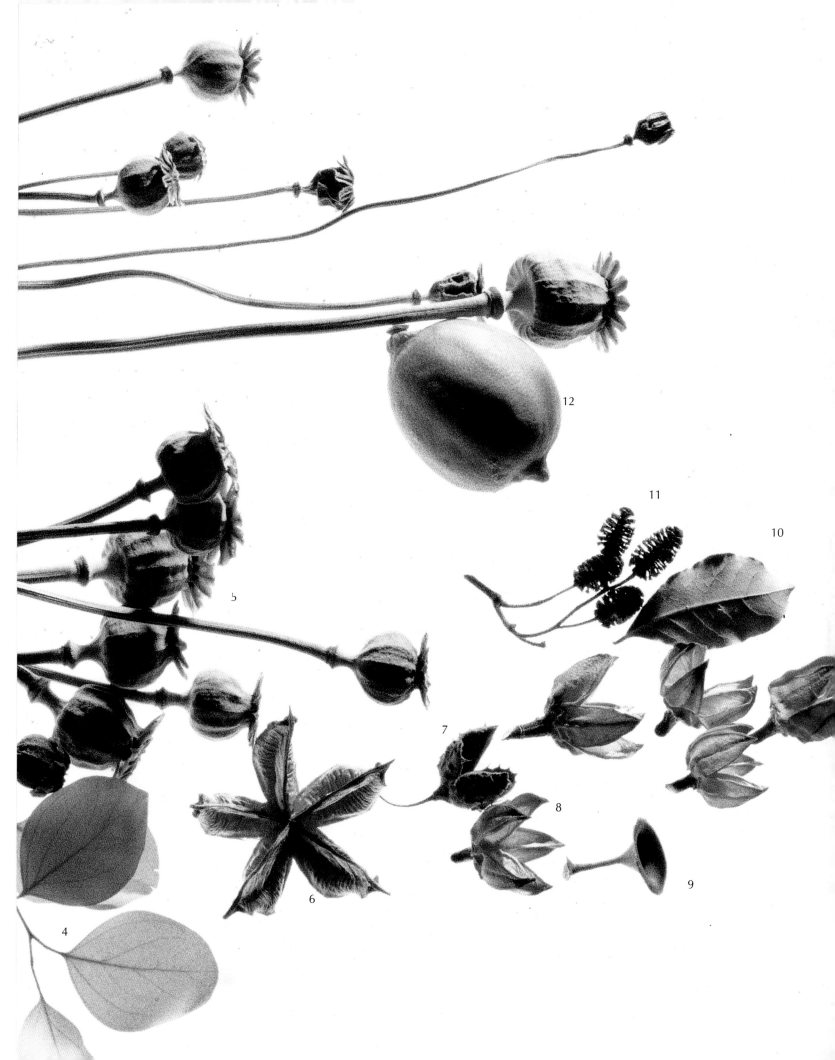

4

5

6

7

8

9

10

11

12

Spices and Fixatives

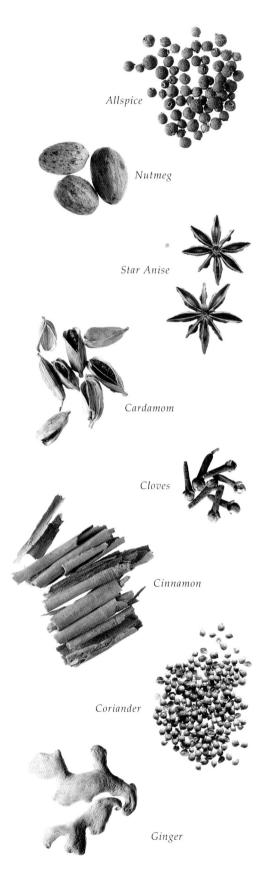

Allspice

Nutmeg

Star Anise

Cardamom

Cloves

Cinnamon

Coriander

Ginger

*M*ost pot-pourri recipes require the addition of some kind of spice to enhance the scents of the rest of the ingredients. The important spices shown here all lend aroma and piquancy.

1. ALLSPICE *Pimenta diocia*

So-called because it smells like a combination of many spices: cloves, juniper berries, cinnamon and pepper. Its spicy, aromatic fragrance blends well with the other classic pot-pourri ingredients, especially lavender, patchouli and orris root.

2. NUTMEG *Myristica fragrans*

When dry, the outer covering of nutmeg produces the brittle, yellowish-brown substance we know as mace, which is often more fragrant than the nutmegs themselves. Nutmeg and mace are often mentioned in old pot-pourri recipes, and are still in use today for their fresh, light, warm fragrance.

3. STAR ANISE *Illicium verum*

From China, this spice is the fruit of a large evergreen tree. Its yellow, narcissus-like flowers are followed by fruits which open into an eight-pointed star and very often the shiny, brown seeds can be seen trapped inside the points of the star. They carry a distinctive aniseed scent.

4. CARDAMOM *Elettaria cardamomum*

Powerfully aromatic, with a pleasing fresh spiciness, cardamom works well not only in spicy pot-pourris but with floral and citrus blends as well, to which it adds an exotic note. After saffron, it is the world's most expensive spice, but is well worth using. You can sometimes buy the empty husks after the small black seeds have been extracted, which are much less costly. The husks are not as fragrant, but carry some residual scent.

5. CLOVES *Eugenia aromatica*

Every part of the clove tree abounds with aromatic oil, but it is the undeveloped flower buds of the tree, which does not fruit until it is eight or nine years old, which we know as cloves. This most useful spice is a fixative and has been valued for centuries for use in perfume and aromatics. Cloves add a dry, uplifting note to both floral and spicy mixes.

6. CINNAMON *Cinnamomum zeylanicum*

Due to its absorbent qualities and tenacious, aromatic scent, cinnamon is useful for adding a spicy note to sweet floral blends; it also works as a fixative. The quills used in aromatics are the dried inner bark of the shoots. Cassia, or Chinese cinnamon, is also useful, but less aromatic. The decorative bark looks good in pot-pourris and its quills are harder and less fragile than true cinnamon, and it is also less expensive.

7. CORIANDER *Coriandrum sativum*

Coriander seed, with its spicy, sweet, rather woody fragrance, is the fruit of an ancient herb. The seeds become increasingly fragrant the longer they are kept. Whole or crushed coriander seeds are very useful in oriental and spicy pot-pourris. Soaked in fragrance, they carry scent well and contribute their own distinctive aroma to a blend.

8. GINGER *Zingiber officinale*

Grown throughout the tropics, the penetrating and aromatic scent of ginger can be effective in a spicy or exotic pot-pourri, but it must be used with great care for it is very powerful. Whole or sliced dried ginger root not only looks good in certain spicy and exotic pot-pourri blends and scented decorations, but contributes just enough of its own distinctive scent to the mix. But beware, do not use too much as it can make you sneeze!

At least one fixative is required for a successful pot-pourri, to absorb the essential oils and impart a distinctive fragrance of its own. Many fixatives are mentioned in old pot-pourri recipes, some with romantic names like Balsam of Peru and Balm of Gilead. Some, like orris root, have an almost magical ability to draw perfumes together and enhance them, and all fixatives hold and maintain the scent of a well-made pot-pourri over a long period of time. Here are some of the most interesting and useful fixatives that are readily available.

1. GUM BENZOIN *Styrax officinalis*

Among the world's oldest perfumes, benzoin carries one of the most pleasant smells of all the gums – a sweet, balsamic note with overtones of vanilla. Like many other resins, it is collected by wounding the bark of the tree and scraping off "almonds" of resin that form on the surface. A strong fixative, it has been used in pot-pourris for centuries.

2. ORRIS ROOT *Iris florentina*

When sliced, chopped or powdered, the root of the Florentine iris carries a faint scent of violets and has a mysterious ability to act as a catalyst in perfume blends, pulling the mix together and enhancing its character. It is lifted, peeled, sliced, dried and then cured for many months before it is fit for use.

3. OAKMOSS *Evernia purpuracea*

A silvery-green lichen which grows on the trunks of oaks and other trees, oakmoss has been used as a perfume ingredient for thousands of years. It is very absorbent, readily taking up and holding the perfumes of other ingredients while imparting its own faint, honeyed scent of new-mown hay.

4. FRANKINCENSE *Boswellia carteri*

Often used in gum form, frankincense was one of the most highly prized substances in ancient times. Its uplifting scent carries a deliciously spicy, woody note and to this day its heavenly fragrance – often combined with myrrh – can be smelled burning in all the great cathedrals of the world.

5. MYRRH *Commiphora myrrha*

This gum resin has a musty, balsamic, incense-like scent and is useful for adding a dry "grounding" note to a pot-pourri.

6. SANDALWOOD *Santalum album*

Thirty years after planting, the essential oil can be extracted from the heartwood of the sandalwood tree and retains its sweet, soft scent almost indefinitely. Every part of the tree is fragrant and even the sawdust is saved and used in sachets and to make joss sticks. The raspings share the delicious aroma said to induce calm and relaxation. This precious wood is a useful fixative for pot-pourris.

7. TONQUIN BEAN *Dipteryx odorata*

These beans are the seeds of *Dipteryx odorata* and they only develop their strong scent once they have been cut from the plant. Very fragrant when fresh, and powerfully fixative, they contain coumarin, which has the aroma of new-mown hay.

8. CALAMUS ROOT *Calamus aromaticus*

All parts of the sweet sedge or flag iris: roots, stems and leaves are fragrant. Native to India, it was first introduced to England in 1596. Calamus has insecticidal properties and a sweet, aromatic smell with a cinnamon-like note. Because of its clean smell, it was used for centuries as a strewing herb. The chopped root is a good fixative and carries perfume through the blend while lending its own subtle fragrance to a pot-pourri mix.

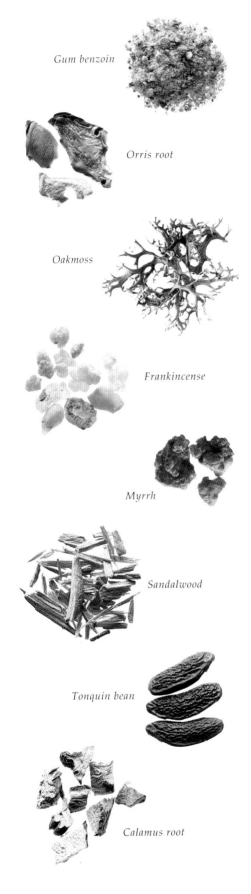

Gum benzoin

Orris root

Oakmoss

Frankincense

Myrrh

Sandalwood

Tonquin bean

Calamus root

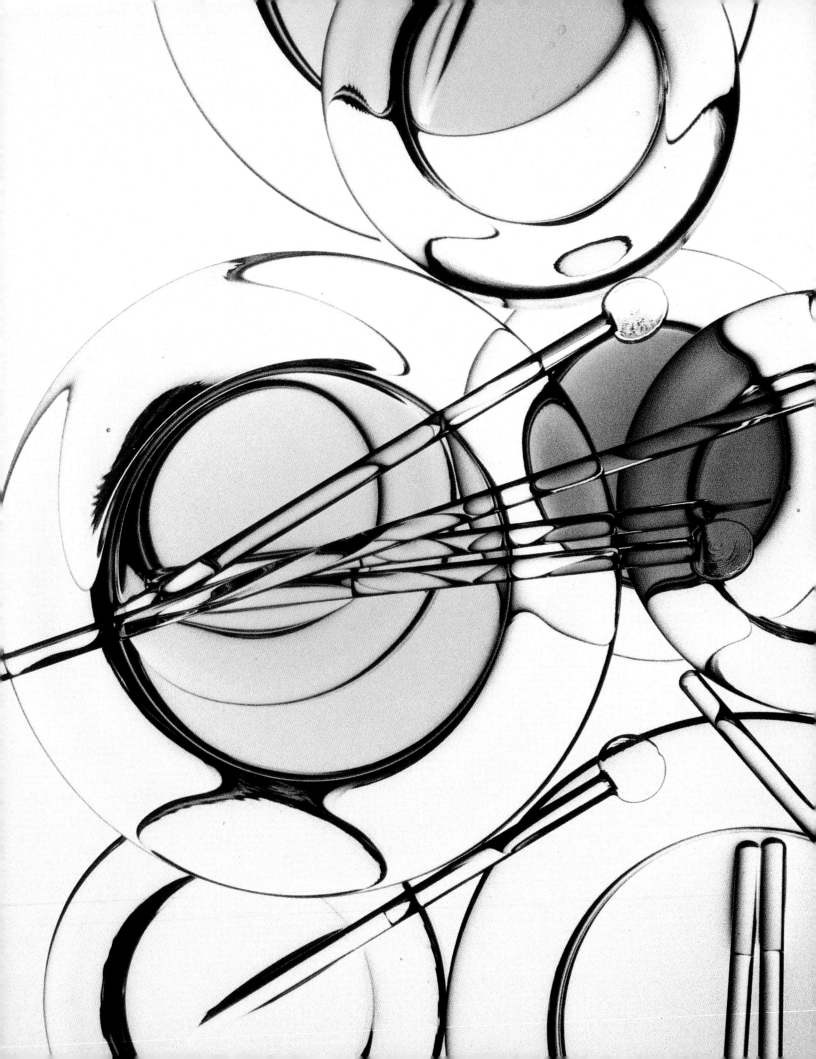

Essential Oils

As long ago as the 2nd century AD, alchemists were extracting the perfume

from plants in a process known as "quintessence." Essential oils as we

know and use them today have their origins in this ancient method of

distilling natural oils from flowers, leaves, barks and roots.

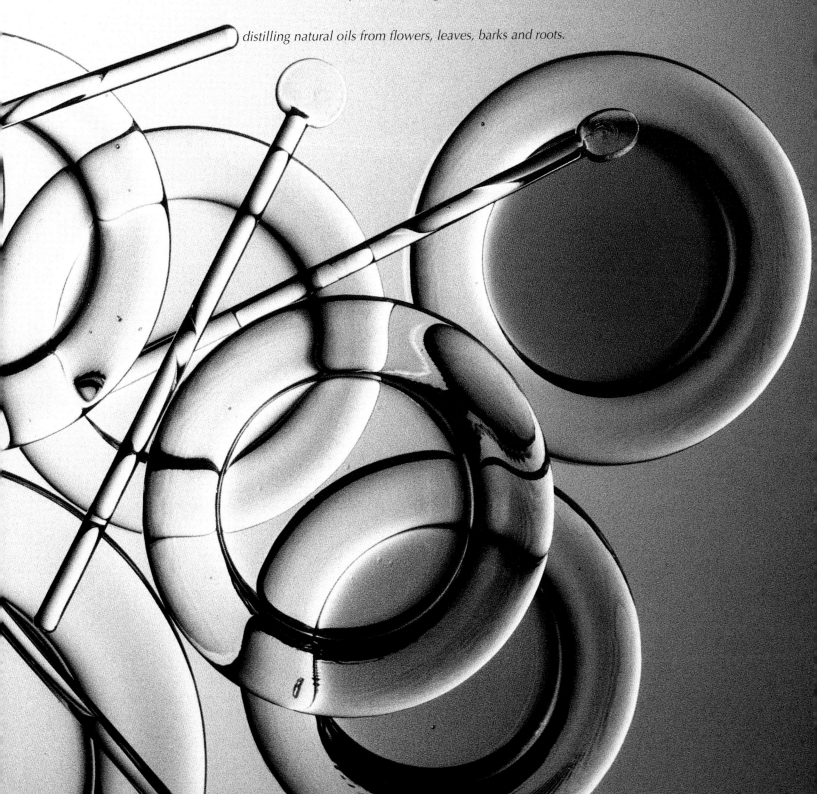

Using Oils

An essential oil is the fragrance which we perceive when we smell a perfumed flower, or press a scented leaf or stem. These magical substances are found in different parts of various plants. For instance, in roses the floral parts are strongly scented; in geraniums it is the leaves; the roots of vetiver and the rhizomes of orris carry most scent. The peels of citrus fruits yield essential oils, and gum resins from some tree barks provide us with oils like frankincense and myrrh. Because there are hundreds of oils available, the following pages illustrate a selection aimed to inspire.

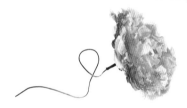

PRICE AND RARITY

Oils are extracted from plants by various methods and all require a great deal of work and a vast number of flowers to produce even the tiniest amount of essential oil. For example, up to 60,000 rose blooms will make just ½oz of essential rose oil (known as otto or absolute.) Essential oils are always measured and sold by weight.

STORAGE

Germicidal qualities in natural oils prevent decay, and as perfume ingredients they keep almost indefinitely. Used therapeutically, most aromatherapists give them a shelf life of about two years. Although pure oils will not go bad or turn rancid, they are affected by ultra-violet rays and so must be protected from sunlight. For this reason you should always store oils and blends in a cool, dark place in colored glass bottles, preferably brown, referred to by suppliers as amber. You should never store oils in metal or plastic containers: metal will taint the oil and essential oils will quite literally melt plastic.

PURCHASE

Always buy 100 percent pure essential oils from a reliable source. Herbalists, health shops and druggists all stock these oils; expect prices to fluctuate from oil to oil. Many natural fragrances have always been synthesized by perfumers for reasons of cost and scarcity, and these synthetic fragrances are widely used in perfumery. The synthetic representation of a single flower essence varies widely: there are, for example, hundreds of different rose-scented oils. Choose an oil you like, to your purpose and to blend with any other oils in the mix. Synthetics and naturals blend well and enhance each other. I use natural oils where possible. Many are no more expensive than synthetics and they have therapeutic qualities which synthetic oils lack. Natural oils have astonishing properties – just to inhale the aroma of a natural oil is beneficial and helps to balance, soothe or invigorate, or combat minor infections.

BLENDING

The art of blending involves balancing a number of different essences to complement each other and form a perfume with a life of its own, where no one scent predominates. Essential oils evaporate at different rates: the fastest are orange and eucalyptus; among the slowest are patchouli and sandalwood; all the other oils lie somewhere in between.

Perfumers divide this scale of evaporation into three parts: top notes, middle notes and base notes. The top note is the scent you first perceive when smelling a perfume. The middle notes form the heart of the blend and the base notes act as fixatives and make the scent last as long as possible. A good blend of oils should contain one or more of all three notes.

Some oils have powerful scents and must be used carefully. For example, patchouli has a strong, pervasive odor and an affinity with lavender, which is milder. Experiment by blending a drop of each oil together; the patchouli will be dominant. Add lavender, drop by drop, until you have a balance that pleases. Make a note of the proportion for future reference to save time – and oil!

To begin blending use narrow strips of blotting paper to try out combinations of scents. Place a drop of each oil on a separate blotter; smell them separately and together to help decide on the blend. You may have to add more drops to some blotters to achieve a balanced scent. To store used blotters for future use, keep each one in a separate cellophane bag. Do not test essential oils on your skin as they can cause irritation.

When blending a new fragrance use a little glass pipette to measure accurately. Work out your blend in drops, and if you want to make a large quantity of oil, translate the drops into fluid ounces.

You may find, after working with scents for a while, that your nose "tires" and you smell very little. It is then time to take a break, or employ the old perfumer's ploy of breathing through a piece of cashmere or fine wool to "clear" the nose. Finally, follow your nose and avoid oils that do not appeal.

OPPOSITE: *Pure essential oils are powerful natural substances distilled from all sorts of plants.*

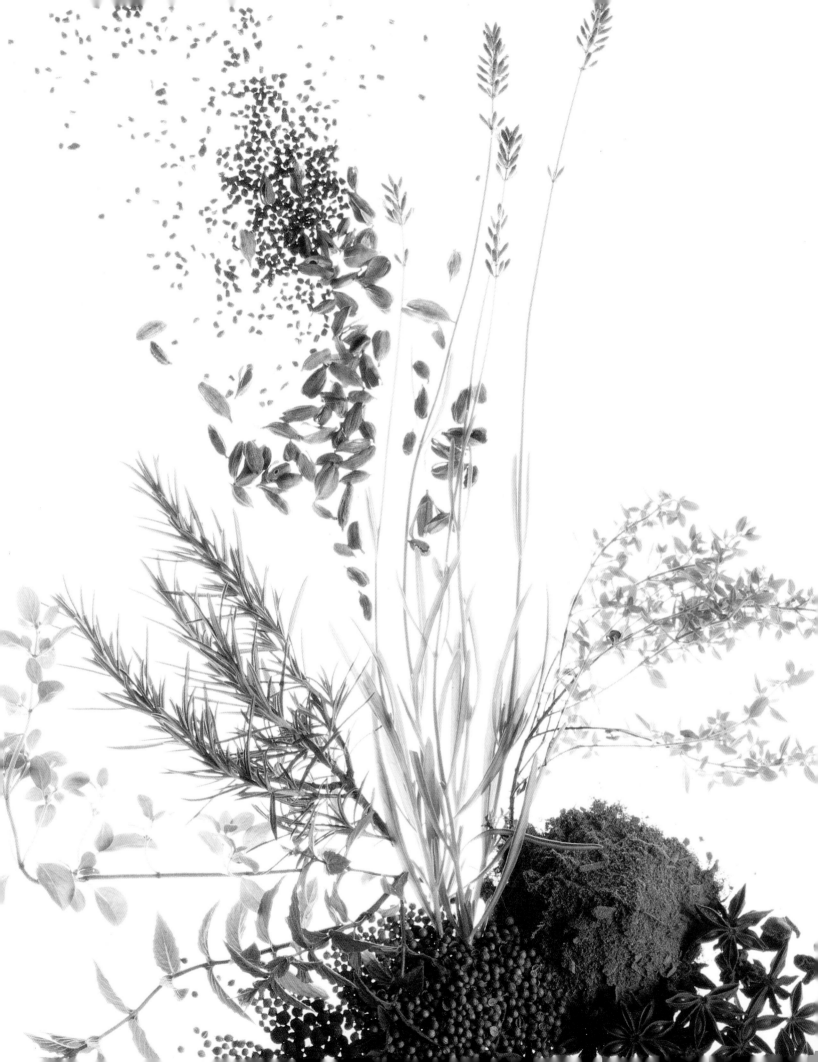

Herb and Spice Oils

Spice and herb oils were once the very cornerstone of perfumery and they continue to be widely used for both fragrance and flavor. Spice oils of one kind or another enter into almost every blend and where a fresh, invigorating note is needed herb oils are invaluable.

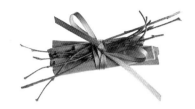

1. ALLSPICE *Pimento dioica*

Contains the aromas of many other spices combined: cloves and juniper berries, black pepper and cinnamon. The oil has a general spicy scent and a fresh top note which blends well with ginger, lavender, rose, patchouli, geranium and orris. Allspice oil has a lovely, fresh, uplifting, spicy scent.

2. CARDAMOM *Elletaria cardamomum*

The pungent seed capsules yield an intensely aromatic oil with a fresh, spicy note. The scent is very pleasant and uplifting and said to help clear the mind. Although expensive, the oil is very potent and should be used with discretion; a little in a blend gives a fresh, spicy note to floral and citrus fragrances.

3. BLACK PEPPER *Piper nigrum*

The berries are picked slightly underripe and sun-dried to give familiar peppercorns which are then distilled to produce an oil with a warm, dry, woody note which blends well with frankincense and sandalwood.

4. CLOVE *Eugenia aromatica*

Cloves are the undeveloped flowerbuds of a small and beautiful evergreen tree, every part of which is aromatic. There are two distinct clove oils – that distilled from the buds (which must be hand-picked) is vastly more expensive than that distilled from the leaves. Reserve clove bud oil for its sweet, spicy note in rosy and floral blends to give a dry note and add richness. Use clove leaf oil in spicy blends and with woody, spicy plant materials.

5. VANILLA *Vanilla planifolia*

Natural vanilla is costly, but there are some less expensive substitutes, such as "vanillin." However, nothing can replace the warm, sweet scent of real vanilla. To make your own vanilla extract take four pods and slit them from end to end. Cut these pieces into sections approximately ¼in long. Place the pieces in an air-tight jar with about 3-5fl oz of high-proof vodka. Soak together for a month; open the jar and shake from time to time. The result is an excellent vanilla extract. The unique rich, warm scent of vanilla acts as a bridge between other perfumes and helps to blend fruits and florals.

6. CINNAMON *Cinnamomum zeylandicum*

The dried inner bark of the young shoots yield the commercial oil, but the shiny, leathery green leaves are distilled for an oil with an aromatic, warm and sweetly spicy scent. Both oils can be used in spicy mixes and blend well with clove and other spice oils.

7. CORIANDER *Coriandrum sativum*

The seeds or fruit of the plant are distilled to produce an oil with a spicy, sweet, slightly woody scent. It blends well with clary sage and lends a spicy-herbal note to rich floral blends of jasmine and lilac.

8. MELISSA *Melissa officinalis*

Although true melissa oil is very costly, it has a unique, delicate herbal scent with delicious lemon overtones. It has an uplifting effect, it soothes and calms and acts as a gentle tonic.

9. THYME *Thymus vulgaris*

This powerfully aromatic herb takes its name from the Greek, *thymos*, which means "to perfume." With its rich, potent, slightly sweet, warm scent, it blends well with other herb oils and citrus perfumes. Useful in all herbal pot-pourris, a tiny quantity of thyme oil combines well with lavender. It has a balancing effect, invigorating where necessary and helping sleep, making it appropriate for use in herb pillows and bath oils.

10. ROSEMARY *Rosmarinus officinalis*

The oil is usually distilled from the whole plant and has a distinctive, penetrating scent. It is one of the most important oils in perfumery and its clean, "piney" notes combine well with lavender, bergamot, basil and all the citrus oils. It makes a refreshing and invigorating "wake-up" bath oil. It is good to burn, or use in a pot-pourri where you work, as it helps to improve memory, hence "rosemary for remembrance." It is useful in all herby pot-pourris and fresh citrus blends.

11. MINT *Mentha piperita* (Peppermint); *Mentha spicata* (Spearmint)

All the mints yield fragrant oils by distillation. Mint oils have the unusual attributes of improving and mellowing with age. Both peppermint and spearmint are used to give "lift" to a blend. Peppermint in particular gives a cool, fresh top note and has a special affinity with lavender, which it enhances when used in very small quantities. These two oils have distinct scents. Spearmint is softer and "mintier" than peppermint which has a drier, peppery note to it and is excellent in cooling summer citrus blends. The softer fragrance of spearmint combines well with herbs and citrus scents in pot-pourris.

OPPOSITE: *A range of herb and spice oils; the numbers relate to the descriptions above.*

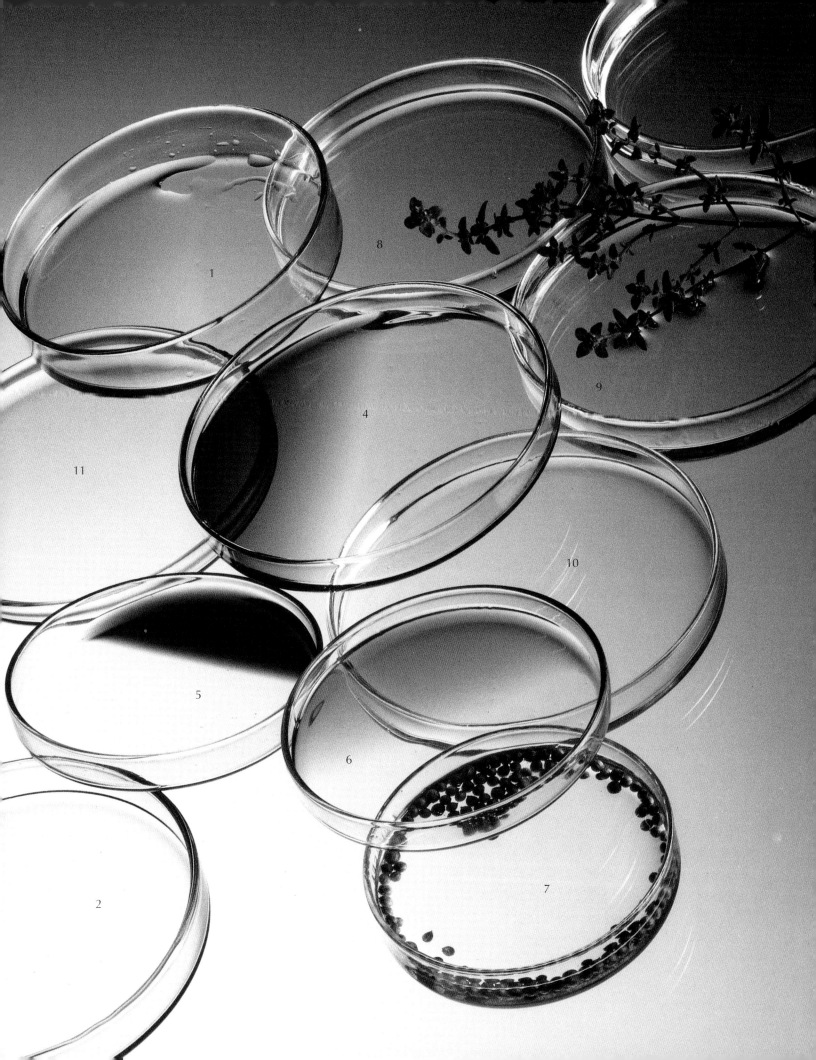

Flower and Fruit Oils

Although the floral oils described here are natural essences and for the most part fairly inexpensive, some of the most famous flower oils such as rose, jasmine and neroli are so costly that it makes their use in pot-pourris and room fragrances quite uneconomic. However, there are all sorts of excellent synthetic oils on the market. Natural fruit-scented oils are inexpensive and they play a part in many different oil blends from spicy, through herby to floral.

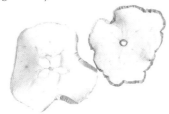

1. ORANGE *Citrus sinensis* (Sweet orange); *Citrus aurantium* (Bitter/Seville orange)

The rich, golden oil of sweet orange seems full of the sun it has soaked up while ripening, and is a wonderful winter oil. It blends well with the spice oils, especially clove and cinnamon, with other citrus oils and works well in herby pot-pourris. Bitter orange oil has the same uses, but a more delicate scent.

2. LAVENDER *Lavandula officinalis*

The flowering tops and stalks of lavender are distilled to produce an oil with a refreshing, floral-herby scent. Lavender has its place in most pot-pourris and aromatics, from herbal, through floral to spicy, woody mixes. It has an affinity with clove and patchouli. The familiar fresh scent of lavender is soothing, calming, balancing and aids sleep.

3. YLANG-YLANG *Cananga odorata*

'Flower of flowers' is the translation of ylang-ylang. These heavily scented cream-colored flowers are distilled for two distinct oils.

There is the finer, intensely floral ylang-ylang with a powerfully sweet fragrance – a scent like mingled jasmine and almonds. And also the heavier, but more tenacious cananga oil, often used in soaps. I often use both oils in rich floral and oriental blends and as a top note in certain rich, woody pot-pourris. The oils have a calming and relaxing effect.

4. BERGAMOT *Citrus bergemia*

Although perhaps the least well-known of the citrus plants, bergamot is by far the most important as a perfume ingredient. The oil comes from the peel and has an extremely rich, fruity top note and a floral, dry-out note, (much used in classic Eau de Cologne). I use bergamot to give a sharp note to sweet florals and a rich, sweet fruity top note to spicy mixes.

5. LEMON GRASS *Cymbopogon citratus*

An oil with a distinct lemon-peel scent. It is very powerful and must be used with care when blending as it can easily swamp other fragrances. It gives an uplifting zing to herby and citrus pot-pourris and adds a sharp note to spicy blends. Cooling and refreshing, it is useful in spring and summer mixes. It also acts as an effective insect repellent, especially when used in combination with lavender.

6. LIME *Citrus aurantifolia*

The most tender of all the citrus oils. West Indian lime oil is cooling and refreshing and blends remarkably well with all the spice oils and some soft oriental oils like patchouli.

7. CHAMOMILE *Ormemsis multicaulis*

An oil with a herbal-fruity fragrance and an intensely floral top note, that is considerably less expensive than German and Roman chamomile oils, which should be reserved for therapeutic purposes. Its distinctive scent is soothing and uplifting.

8. GERANIUM *Pelargonium graveolens*

This beautiful oil has an intensely flowery scent which is so like rose that it is widely used in rosy-floral mixes. Used in small amounts it will blend with almost any other oil, acting as a catalyst by drawing together other fragrances and lending its own slightly green, floral quality to the whole blend. I often use geranium in floral and herby mixes, and it also blends well with the citrus oils.

9. PALMAROSA *Cymbopogon martini*

This important oil is relatively inexpensive and widely used in the perfume industry. The leaves and stems are processed to yield an oil with an amazingly rich, sweet, rosy-floral fragrance somewhere between geranium and rose, with a slightly lemony undertone. A lovely scent in its own right, I use it to lend natural freshness to synthetic rose perfumes.

10. GRAPEFRUIT *Citrus x paradisi*

The thick, golden-yellow peel of grapefruit produces a distinctively sharp and refreshing oil. Small amounts of grapefruit blend well with many of the spice oils and soft exotics such as patchouli and sandalwood to produce a citrus-spicy scent for pot-pourri. For long-distance travel this invigorating oil is a valuable aid in combating jetlag.

11. PETITGRAIN *Citrus bigaradia*

The word petitgrain translates as "little seeds." The oil was once produced from the tiny unripe fruits of the bitter orange tree. Today the oil is more economically derived from the leaf tips and young shoots, but the name remains. The blossom of the same tree give us neroli, one of the world's most costly oils. Petitgrain has a fresh, light, flowery perfume and its uplifting scent blends well with rosemary, lavender, geranium and bergamot.

OPPOSITE: *An array of floral and fruit oils; the numbers correspond to the descriptions above.*

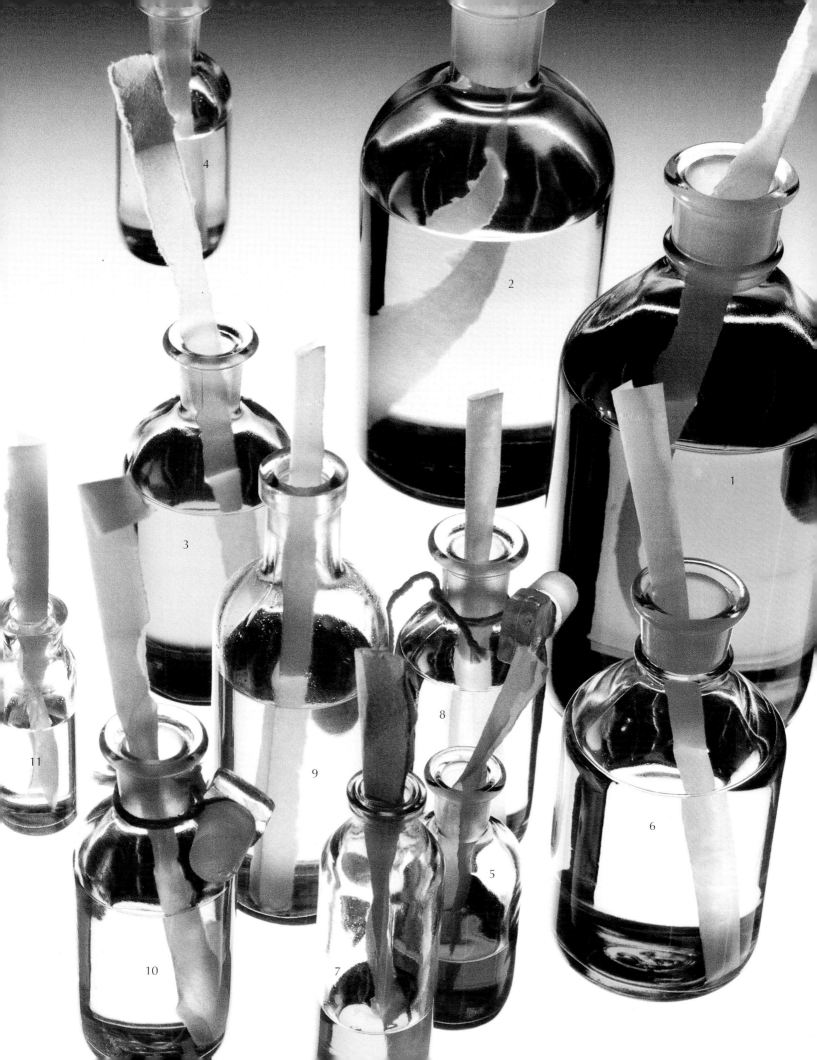

Gums and Balsam Oils

These oils are all strongly fixative and number among them some of the most pleasing perfumes known to man. Vetiver is included in this group both for its fixative qualities and its unique earthy scent, although it is neither a gum nor a balsam, being distilled from the roots of a scented grass. The fixative oils play an essential role in every blend. Not always obviously perfumed scents in their own right, they are nevertheless tenacious and have the ability to draw other scents together and enhance the blend.

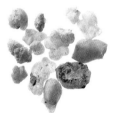

1. LABDANUM *Cistus ladaniferum*

An oil with an extremely sweet and agreeable warm, honey-like, musky scent which is soothing and balsamic. It is widely used in perfumes and expensive soaps. It has a richness and depth all of its own and blends wonderfully with many other oils, often adding that indefinable something to a blend.

2. BENZOIN *Styrax benzoin*

Often referred to as Benjamin or Oil of Ben in old recipes. The resin is extracted by deliberately wounding the tree bark which exudes a reddish-brown resinoid or "absolute." Benzoin has a sweet, balsamic note that is reminiscent of vanilla and blends especially well with rose and sandalwood. It is one of the most useful fixative oils and helps to fix scent for many months, even years. I use it in many blends as its sweet, warm, vanilla balsam scent is equally happy in both floral and spicy blends.

3. GALBANUM *Ferula galbaniflu*

The Babylonians knew the powerfully "green" smell of galbanum and used it as incense thousands of years ago. It is an oil with a potent, green, woody fragrance, it is strongly fixative and often used by perfumers in pine and mossy blends. This extraordinary oil has a fascinating "ancient" quality. Use it in tiny quantities, or it will completely take over.

4. STORAX *Liquidambar orientalis*

A semi-fluid balsam with the consistency of honey, storax has an agreeable vanilla-like aroma and is strongly fixative. I find oils such as storax useful as an effective fixative where a balsamic, warm, spicy note is called for in a blend, be it floral or spicy. Note that storax can also be referred to as styrax.

5. VETIVER *Vetiveria zizanoides*

The rhizomes of this plant yield a viscous oil with a pungent scent reminiscent of roots, soil and wood. It has a distinctive, fresh fragrance and powerful fixative qualities, acting as a catalyst in a blend by enhancing and drawing together all the other scents. It can provide an earthy base note in potpourri and burning-oil blends. It is especially useful when a mix of fragrances is "flying away" and requires "earthing." It blends well with sandalwood and jasmine.

6. BALSAM OF PERU *Myroxylon balsamum*

Often mentioned in old recipes, this tree is not in fact from Peru but originates in El Salvador, from where Peruvian goods (including this balsam) were shipped to Europe, hence its romantic name. Every part of the tree is aromatic and the flowers can be smelled from 100 yards away. The oil has a thick, viscous, honey-like texture and a rich, soft, sweet and tenacious perfume. It is an excellent fixative. Because of its consistency small quantities are usually sold in little jars. The Tolu tree is a related tree that yields the similar balsam of Tolu, which has a more refined scent than balsam of Peru. Balsam of Tolu is sold in pots or jars; it sets quite hard and must be heated to liquefy it.

7. FRANKINCENSE *Boswellia carteri*

The name frankincense has become synonymous with incense and in France it is simply known as *"encens."* One of the first gums to be burnt as incense, it has been in constant use since earliest antiquity. The Egyptian pharoah-queen Hatshepsut mounted a famous expedition to the land of Punt to bring back frankincense trees to adorn her temple at Thebes. The walls of the temple are decorated with a wonderful series of carvings depicting the expedition with detailed representations of the trees and their roots bound up for transportation. Frankincense has an uplifting scent and gives a splendid top note to various blends, in particular the rich, spicy mixes of the winter season. It can also give lift and a dry note to exotic floral blends.

8. MYRRH *Commiphora myrrha*

The tree grows in hot, dry climates and secretes a gum which hardens and is scraped off and distilled to yield an essential oil which blends happily with frankincense. The two have been inextricably linked since earliest times. Myrrh and frankincense are burnt together to produce the heavenly scent found in all the great cathedrals of the world. Myrrh is not a sweet scent: it has a musty, slightly bitter, smoky-balsamic smell which adds a dry grounding note to a blend. Used with discretion it adds an indefinable touch of mystery to oriental and rich, spicy blends.

OPPOSITE: *A selection of gum and balsam oils; the numbers relate to the descriptions above.*

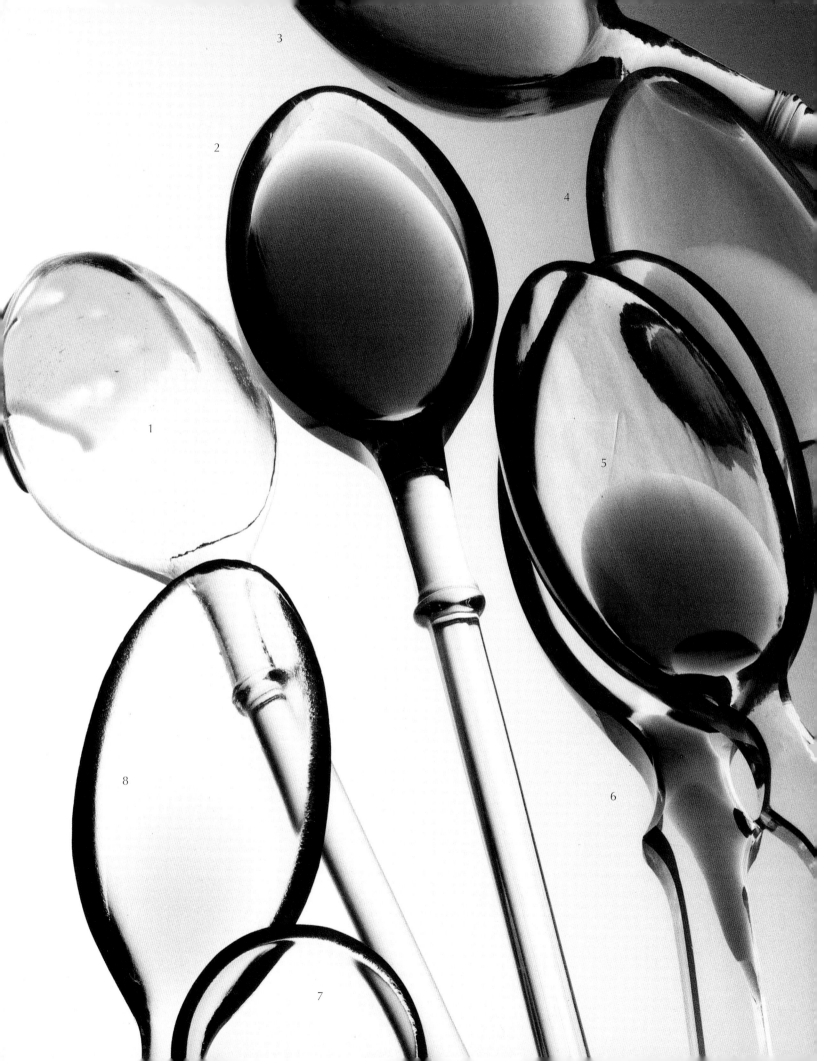

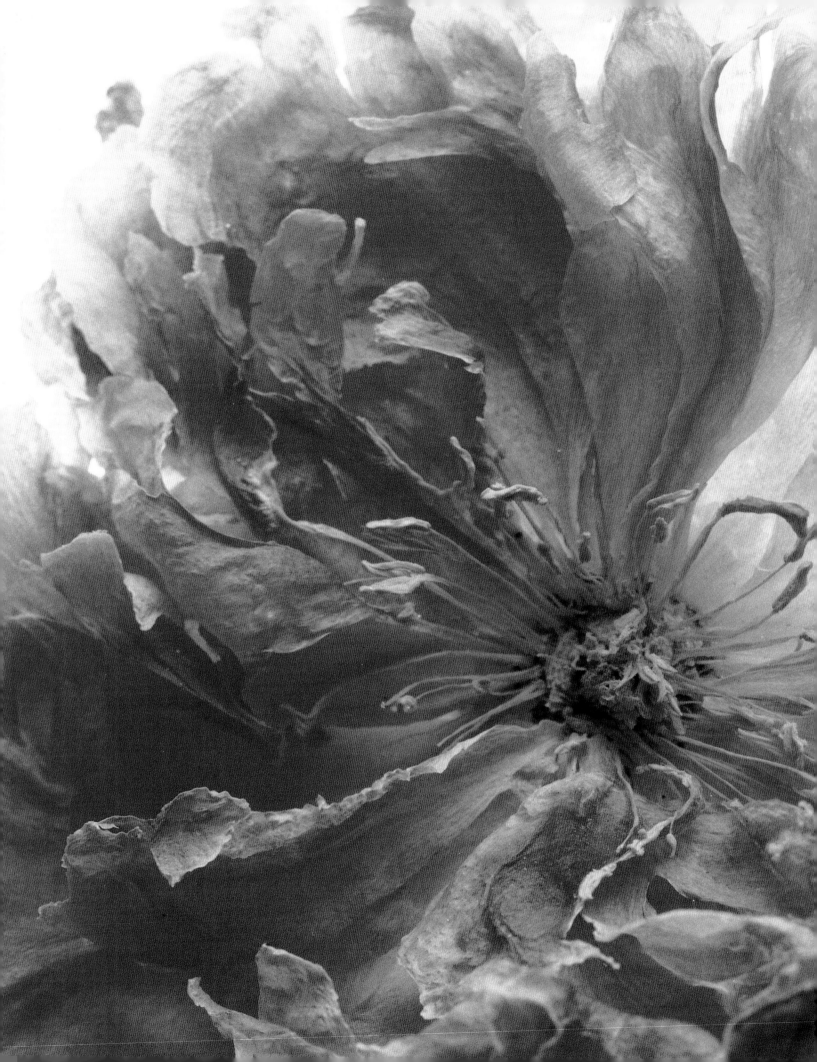

POT-POURRIS

ALTHOUGH READY-MADE POT-POURRIS ARE EASY TO OBTAIN,

THE INGREDIENTS USED IN COMMERCIALLY PRODUCED MIXES

ARE OFTEN OF POOR QUALITY AND MAKE USE OF FAIRLY

UNINSPIRING PLANT MATERIALS. BY PREPARING YOUR OWN

POT-POURRIS YOU CAN VASTLY EXTEND THE SCOPE OF DRIED

SCENTED FLOWERS AND HERBS, SPICES AND AROMATICS.

WITH THE WEALTH OF PLANT MATERIAL AVAILABLE TODAY

ALL YOU NEED IS THE INCLINATION AND A LITTLE TIME TO

SPARE TO PRODUCE ENDLESS VARIATIONS OF POT-POURRIS BY

EITHER THE MOIST OR THE DRY METHOD.

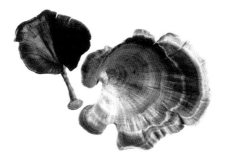

Moist Pot-Pourri Making

Traditional moist pot-pourris were made according to family recipes that were often adapted to suit what was to hand. Highly scented rose petals were usually the main ingredients, along with other fragrant flowers, aromatic leaves and herbs. These were partially dried and layered with coarse salt (which acted as a preservative) in a glazed earthenware pot. The mixture was then left to mature until it "caked" into a compacted mass. The "cake" was removed from the pot, broken up and perfumed with the addition of spices, fixatives and oils. The pot-pourri was then placed in a covered jar and set to "cure" for at least eight weeks until ready for use; some recipes advocate curing for between six months and a year. The resulting mix was not attractive to look at, although it smelled quite wonderful. The pot-pourri was kept in china containers, often of great beauty and value, with a pierced or fretted inner lid, covered by a solid outer lid. The containers stood on a chimney-piece or a table near the fireplace; when the fire was lit the outer lid was removed and the fragrance of the pot-pourri allowed to escape into the room. To make the traditional pot-pourris on pages 50-56 follow the method given here, which is quite simple and involves no stirring, pouring away of liquid or daily turning. The photographs that accompany the recipes are in the style of the picture opposite and show the decorative trimmings and some salient ingredients that should lie on top of the finished mix; the pictures aim to give a clear idea of the unique character of each pot-pourri.

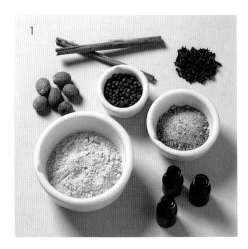

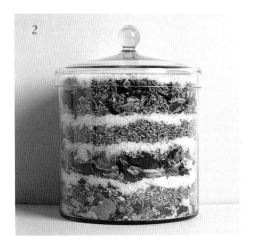

1. Collect a quantity of scented roses, which must be absolutely dry when picked. Strip off the petals, separate them and lay them out to semi-dry on frames (see page 26) or spread over a cloth on the floor. The petals will lose about half their bulk during the semi-drying process. The time this takes depends upon temperature and atmospheric conditions, but is usually about two days. The petals are ready when they have a tough, leathery texture. Coarse salt is added to preserve the petals and prevent mold. In the past, a mix of bay salt and common salt was used. Bay salt is sometimes available, but if not use pure sea or kosher salt. Never use iodized salt.

Place a layer of dried plant material in the bottom of a straight-sided glass or glazed earthenware jar. Cover this with a layer of salt. Press down with a circle of cardboard cut to fit inside the circumference of the jar mouth, or use a small plate. Old pot-pourri jars had a special leaded weight for this purpose. The first layer of dried plant material in the base of the jar should be approximately ½in deep when pressed down. Cover the layer of petals with a good sprinkling of salt. Repeat the layering until the jar is full. You can add more layers of petals as they become available; always end with a layer of salt.

Soft leaves, such as scented geranium, should be torn into shreds and dried in the same way as the rose petals; likewise other scented flowers. Material of a dry nature such as lavender, rosemary and bay leaves can be added to the jar just as they are, without completing the semi-drying process.

2. Keep the mixture packed down inside the jar for at least six weeks. Here I have used a glass jar so that you can see the layers. If you choose a glass container, keep it in a dark place while the mixture matures. When it is ready it will be compacted into a "cake." Pre-prepare a mix of spices, fixatives and oils together in a small bowl. Remove the "cake" from the jar and break it up into small pieces in a large mixing bowl. Add the mixed spices, fixatives and oils to the broken-up "cake." Always stir with a wooden spoon as perfumes are affected by contact with metal. The potency of scent is a personal matter and it is best to add perfume little by little; you can always add to a scent but it is impossible to tone it down. Note that the scent tends to strengthen as the pot-pourri matures.

Press the scented mixture tightly back into the jar, cover and leave to mature for at least a further two months – the longer it is left to cure, the better the finished result will be.

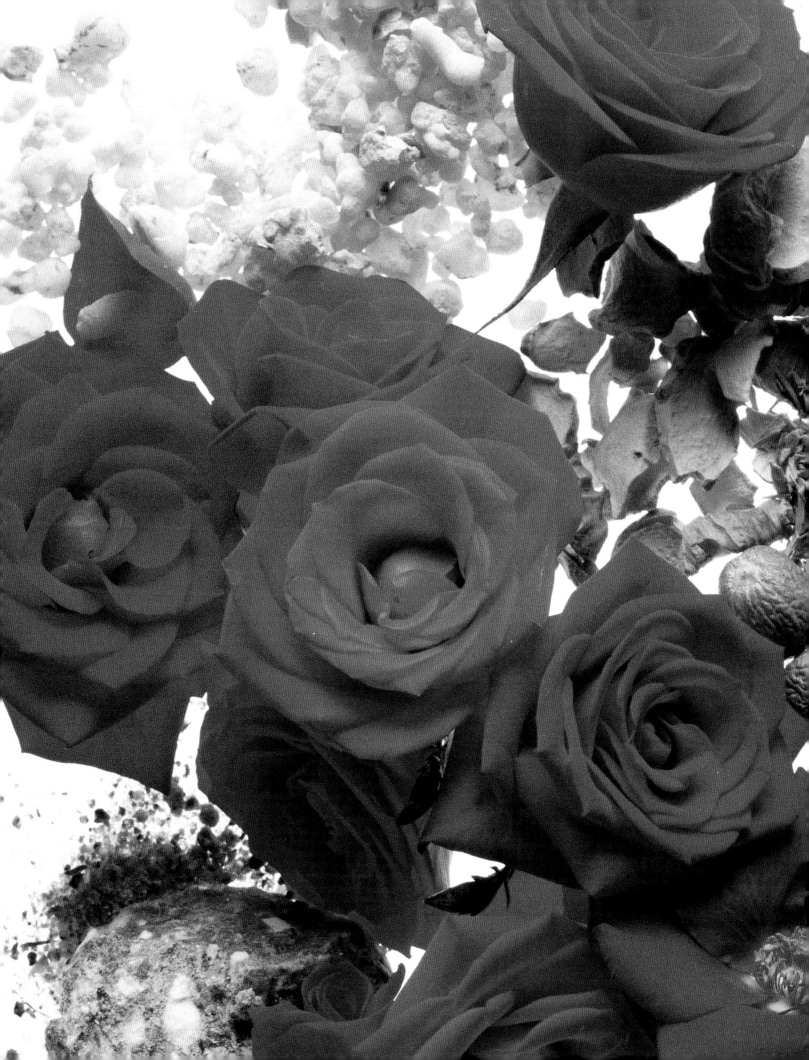

Aunt Beth's and Derbyshire Rose Pot-Pourris

Here are two pot-pourri recipes that have been handed down in my family. I adapted the original recipes which contained animal fixatives such as musk and ambergris, that are no longer available. A small amount of clary sage oil has been added: this oil is said to be the closest fragrance to ambergris.

For Aunt Beth's pot-pourri, because modern rose varieties are not so fragrant as those used when the mix was first concocted, I greatly increased the amount of rose-scented oil in my adaptation. The original recipe specified just a few drops of attar or otto of rose oil, which is now prohibitively expensive.

All sorts of varieties of the fragrant Rosa gallica and Rosa centifolia were used in pot-pourri making in the past, but Derbyshire Rose was probably made with the dark red Rosa gallica officinalis or 'Provins' rose which is one of the world's most fragrant roses and was grown in Derbyshire for medicinal purposes up until the 1920's.

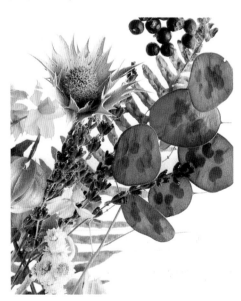

AUNT BETH'S POT-POURRI

Here I used violet-scented oil instead of rose geranium, as the latter can develop an odd smell as it ages. Follow the method on page 48.

THE INGREDIENTS
THE BASE PLANTS
1lb 8oz semi-dry rose petals

12oz semi-dry fragrant flower mix: stock, heliotrope, mignonette, jasmine etc

4oz lavender flowers

8oz mix of semi-dry torn leaves: rose-scented geranium, sweet verbena, rosemary and lemon thyme

THE FIXATIVES
1lb coarse sea salt

2oz powdered orris root

1oz powdered gum benzoin

THE SPICES
1oz broken cinnamon sticks

1oz whole cloves

THE OILS
140 drops rose-scented (synthetic)

140 drops bergamot

100 drops lemon

80 drops violet-scented (synthetic)

60 drops lavender

40 drops patchouli

20 drops clove

20 drops clary sage

THE TRIMMINGS
Green honesty seedpods

Shoo fly seedpods

White eryngiums (air dried)

Lavender

Polypody fern (pressed)

Anaphalis (air dried)

Juniper berries

Jonquils (silica dried)

DERBYSHIRE ROSE

Condense the method for making moist pot-pourris on page 48 to just one stage. First mix the spices, fixatives and blended oils with sea salt and sprinkle this mixture on to the layers of rose petals; end with a salt and spice layer. Press down tightly, cover and leave to mature for two to three months. If any liquid forms in the bottom of the jar you should pour it off.

THE INGREDIENTS
THE BASE PLANTS
3lb semi-dry rose petals

THE FIXATIVES
1lb coarse sea salt, or other non-iodized salt

4oz sandalwood raspings

4oz chopped dry calamus root

2oz powdered orris root

2oz gum benzoin

1oz gum storax

THE SPICES
2oz chopped dry angelica root

2oz crushed cinnamon sticks

2oz crushed cloves

1oz crushed cardamom seeds

THE OILS
300 drops rose-scented (synthetic)

200 drops sandalwood

100 drops clary sage

THE TRIMMINGS
Open, old-fashioned roses (air dried)

Sprays of pink peppercorns (air dried)

Philadelphus leaves (air dried)

Hydrangea (air dried)

Lavender seeds

Small poppy seedheads

Licheny twig

Whole cloves

ABOVE LEFT: *Trimmings for Aunt Beth's pot-pourri.* OPPOSITE: *Top dressing for the Derbyshire Rose pot-pourri.*

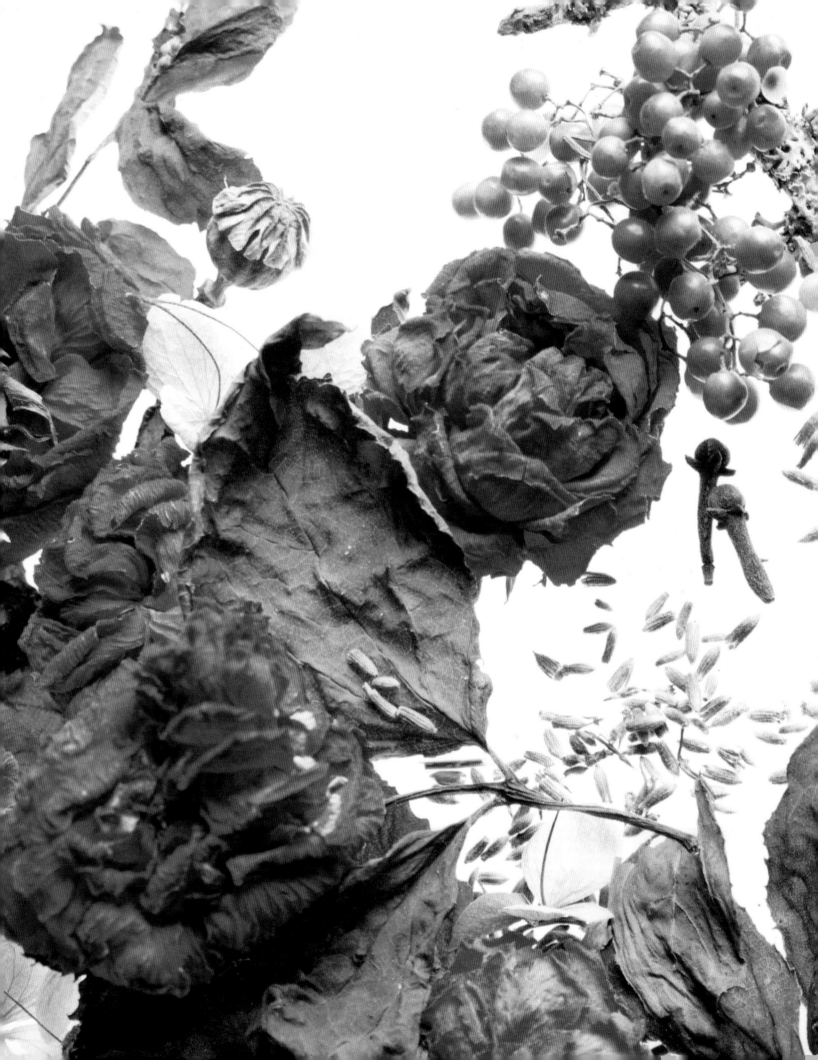

Chelsea and Persian Garden Pot-Pourris

My herby Chelsea mix pays tribute to the Chelsea Physic Garden, founded by the English Society of Apothecaries of London in 1673. The garden was established as a botanical laboratory where physicians and apothecaries studied the medicinal properties of plants. Today, this beautiful walled garden is open to the public and provides an oasis in the heart of London. To reflect the nature of the plants grown at Chelsea I have chosen materials for the mix which belie the usual flowery look of a pot-pourri, such as fern, moss, seedheads and a small dried artichoke head.

By contrast, the Persian Garden mix is a richly scented blend of roses and other fragrant flowers, combined with balsamic fixatives and exotic essential oils to evoke the opulence of an oriental garden. The Persian love of gardens can be seen in their art and woven into rugs; if you have a Persian rug try taking inspiration from the rich colors and designs to concoct your own pot-pourri.

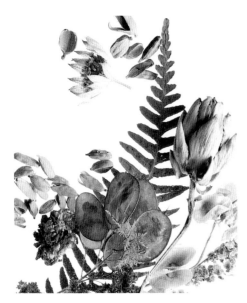

CHELSEA

An invigorating pot-pourri with a herby base inspired by 16th- and 17th-century recipes for strewing herbs. To make, see page 48.

THE INGREDIENTS
THE BASE PLANTS

2lb semi-dry fragrant rose petals

1lb mix of semi-dry fragrant flowers: wallflowers, jonquils, stock etc

8oz semi-dry leaf mix: melissa, sweet geranium and mint

4oz lavender flowers

6oz mix of dried herbs: thyme, rosemary and marjoram

THE FIXATIVES

1lb coarse sea salt

4oz chopped dry calamus root

2oz powdered orris root

THE SPICES

2oz crushed coriander seeds

1oz crushed cloves

½oz powdered allspice

(½o) powdered nutmeg

THE OILS

140 drops lavender

100 drops palmarosa

80 drops geranium

40 drops rosemary

40 drops lemon grass

THE TRIMMINGS

Bells of Ireland (glycerined)

Marjoram

Cardamom pods

Honesty seedpods

Polypody fern (pressed)

Purple double stock (air dried)

Green moss

Miniature artichokes

PERSIAN GARDEN

A richly scented blend of roses and fragrant flowers combined with balsamic fixatives and exotic oils. To make, see page 48.

THE INGREDIENTS
THE BASE PLANTS

2lb 8oz semi-dry rose petals

8oz semi-dry fragrant flowers: heliotrope, jasmine, mignonette etc

4oz lavender flowers

4oz semi-dry torn rose-scented geranium leaves

1oz torn bay leaves

THE FIXATIVES

1lb coarse sea salt

4oz sandalwood raspings

2oz chopped dry angelica root

2oz powdered orris root

½oz powdered gum benzoin

½oz powdered gum storax

THE SPICES

1oz crushed cardamom seeds

½oz powdered allspice

½oz powdered cloves

THE OILS

160 drops palmarosa

100 drops patchouli

60 drops lavender

60 drops cedarwood

20 drops clove, preferably bud

THE TRIMMINGS

Eucalyptus leaves and flowers (air dried)

Bougainvillea (air dried)

Zinnias (silica dried)

Hellebores (silica dried)

Purple astrantia (air dried)

Hydrangea (air dried)

Lavender

ABOVE LEFT: *Top dressing for the Chelsea pot-pourri.* OPPOSITE: *Plant material to trim the Persian Garden pot-pourri.*

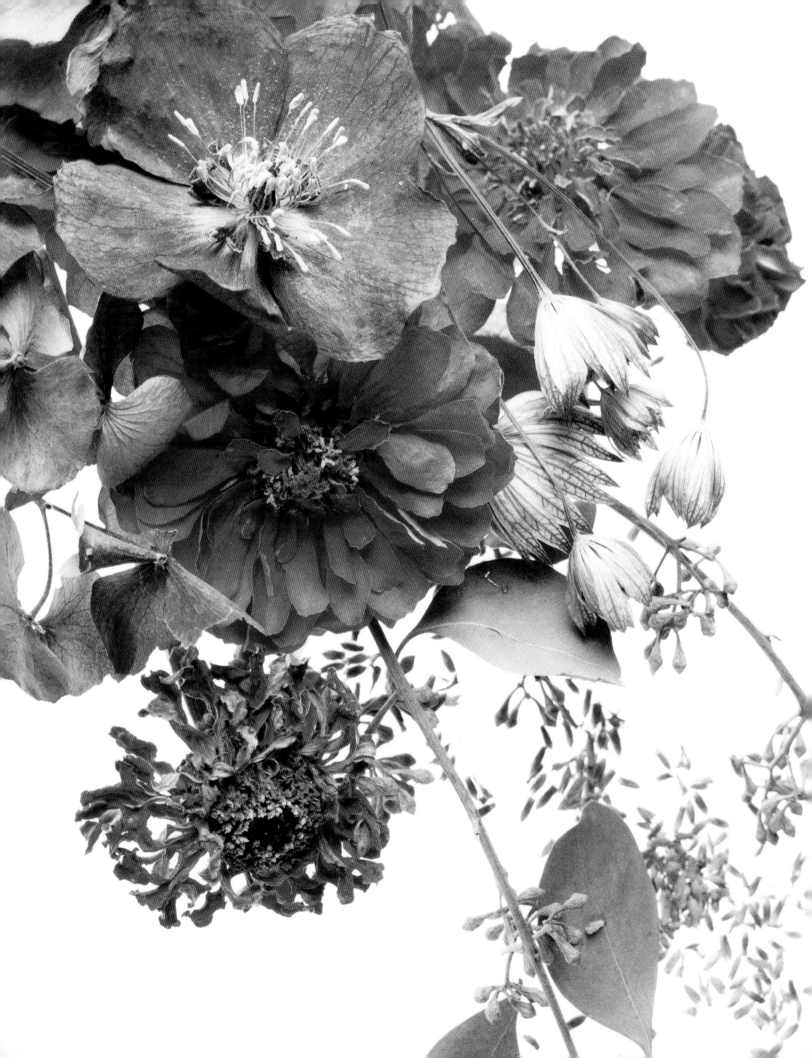

Festival and Bourbon Vanilla Pot-Pourris

The Festival pot-pourri is composed of traditional oils, spices, fruits and gums and the top dressing complements the spicy, fruity scent of the blend of essential oils. The pomegranates lend an interesting touch; you can gild them or impregnate them with oils to spice up the overall fragrance of the mix. If you cannot obtain some of the ingredients in these or any of the previous recipes then always feel free to improvize.

Bourbon Vanilla is a sweet, spicy fall pot-pourri with a fruity top note based on vanilla. Native to Mexico, vanilla is extracted from the dried bean of an orchid. When the orchid was introduced to the Island of Reunion it would not pollinate naturally and, in 1841, the present method of pollinating by hand was perfected. The old name for Reunion is Bourbon and the island still produces the finest vanilla which has a warm, tenacious scent that gives depth to floral pot-pourris and blends well with exotic woods and spices.

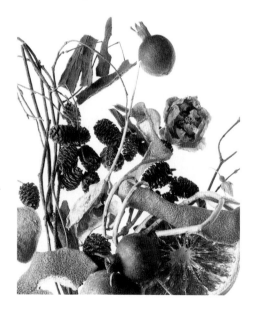

FESTIVAL

A wonderfully warm, rich winter pot-pourri composed from traditional oils, spices, fruits and gums. To make, see page 48.

THE INGREDIENTS
THE BASE PLANTS
2lb 8oz semi-dry fragrant rose petals
in yellow or pale tones
4oz mix of torn semi-dry leaves:
eucalyptus, bay and fresh pine needles

THE FIXATIVES
1lb coarse sea salt
2oz chopped dried orange peel
2oz powdered orris root
2oz powdered gum benzoin

THE SPICES
2oz crushed cinnamon sticks
2oz crushed coriander seeds
1oz crushed cloves
1oz powdered allspice
½oz ground nutmeg

THE OILS
100 drops orange
60 drops frankincense
60 drops bergamot
60 drops cedarwood
40 drops cinnamon
40 drops clove
40 drops myrrh

THE TRIMMINGS
Birch and hazel twigs
Orange peel and pomegranates (air dried)
Orange slices (radiator dried)
Cassia bark
Alder cones
Iris foetidissima seedhead (air dried)
White camellia (silica dried)
Yellow rose buds (air dried)

BOURBON VANILLA

The dominant scent of this pot-pourri is a delicious sweet vanilla, with a touch of orange zest. To make, see page 48.

THE INGREDIENTS
THE BASE PLANTS
3lb semi-dry fragrant rose petals
in yellow and cream
(Avoid using red blooms)
4oz semi-dry torn rose-scented
geranium leaves

THE FIXATIVES
1lb coarse sea salt
2oz powdered orris root
1oz powdered gum benzoin
1oz powdered gum storax
1oz chopped dried orange peel
(Use the thin, outer rind removed with a
sharp paring knife or potato peeler)

THE SPICES
1oz whole coriander seeds
½oz powdered allspice
½oz crushed cloves
½oz crushed cinnamon sticks

THE OILS
100 drops benzoin
100 drops vanilla-scented (synthetic)
80 drops bois de rose
60 drops clove
60 drops orange
40 drops cinnamon

THE TRIMMINGS
Bleached poppy seedheads
Bells of Ireland (glycerined)
Ornamental corn cob
Sponge mushroom and canella berries
Cream eucalyptus leaves (bleached
and glycerined)

ABOVE LEFT: The top dressing for the Festival pot-pourri. OPPOSITE: Plant material to trim the Bourbon Vanilla pot-pourri.

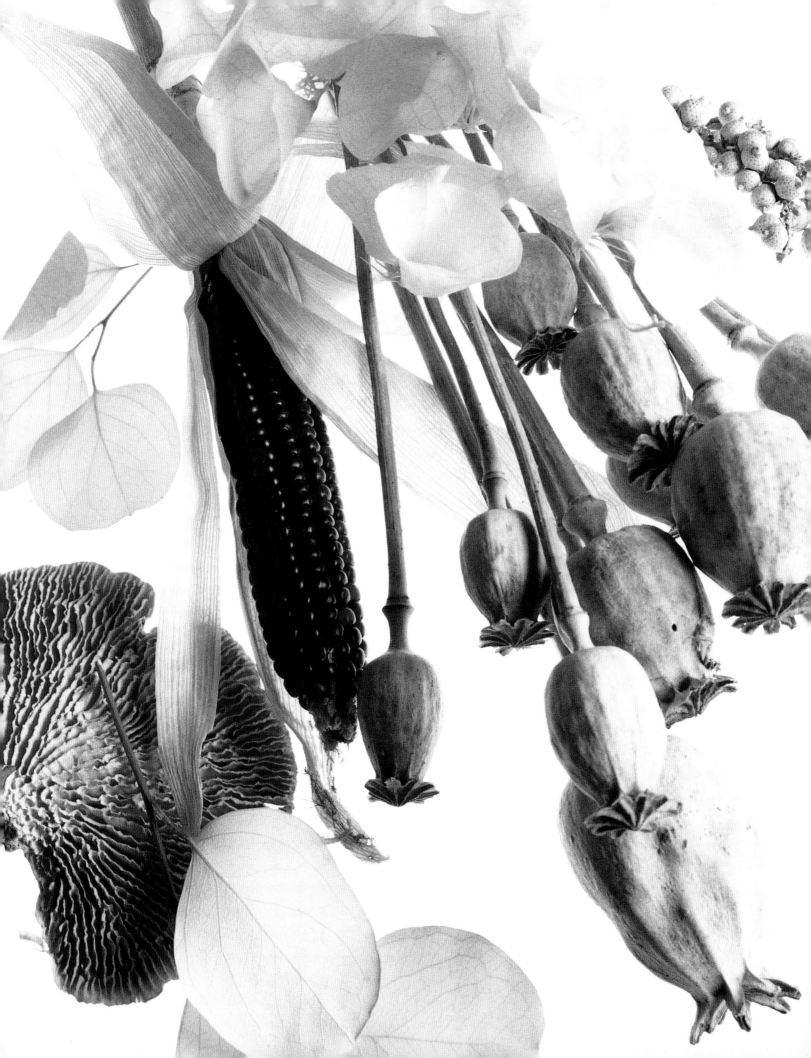

Dry Pot-Pourri Making

I prefer to make pot-pourri using the dry method. It is more straightforward than the traditional moist method given on page 48 and quicker to execute. So long as you use sufficient essential oils and fixatives then the results are as satisfying, long lasting and equally fragrant.

To produce the recipes given on pages 60-88 follow the method explained here. In each recipe the base plants constitute the main body of the pot-pourri. The oils must be blended together rather than added one by one. The powders consist of ground spices and fixatives which will contribute their own scent to the mix and help prolong the overall aroma. The oils and powders combine to form minute scented particles which filter through the mix and distribute their properties. I make dry pot-pourris using all-important carrier materials. These consist of whole spices, seeds and pods which are coated in a blend of perfumed oils and so quite literally transport their scent. Finally, the trimmings describe a top dressing of decorative plant material reserved to enhance the visual effect of the finished pot-pourri. Unlike the moist method, where the trimmings are simply placed on the scented base, here they may also be scented. Do not scent dark-colored trimmings with powders, simply polish them with the oil blend. The photographs accompanying the recipes represent the trimmings and are in the style of the picture opposite. Add the trimmings as a top layer to the finished pot-pourri mix. If some of the ingredients are hard to obtain you may substitute them for alternative plant materials of your choice.

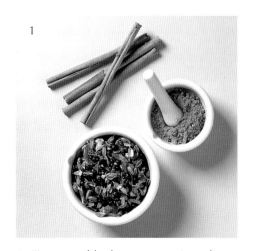

1. First assemble the necessary ingredients. Start with the essential oils. The best way to make a blend of oils is to measure out the specified quantities with care and accuracy into a small, screw-top bottle. Work with the use of a small pipette, counting out the oil in drops. Once you have measured out the necessary oils shake the bottle well to make a blend. Next put the powdered materials, in other words the ground spices and the fixatives, into a small bowl (as seen in the picture above in the right-hand bowl) and mix them together using a small wooden spoon. Then, with a dropper add a very small quantity of the blended oil to the powders and stir until they form a dry, crumbly mix. Add the rest of the blended oils to the carrier materials (as seen in the picture above in the left-hand bowl.) Cover the carrier materials and leave for 24 hours to allow the fragrance to be fully absorbed. If you are using very dark-colored base plant materials you may wish to avoid scenting them with powders as they will turn dusty. Dark-hued trimmings will maintain their natural luster if you just coat them with the blended oils using a paint brush or a Q-tip; in this way they will also help to carry some scent.

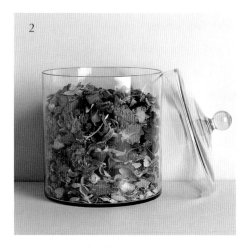

2. Assemble the base plant materials in a large mixing bowl, preferably made of china. A plastic bowl will suffice but note that the plastic may also absorb the fragrance. Here I have shown the base plant ingredients in a glass container, for clarity. Gently mix the base plants together with a wooden spoon until they are well distributed. Then scatter the saturated carrier materials over the base material mix in the large bowl and again turn gently to distribute them evenly. Repeat the process after you have added the crumbly powder mix. Set the scented base materials to mature in a suitable container. This should be large enough to hold the base mix as well as the trimmings which provide a decorative top dressing and are a final addition. Choose china or glass jars for maturing; avoid plastic containers which allow the fragrance to escape, and metal, which may taint the scent. The very fine nylon bags that are sold in supermarkets for roasting poultry are excellent and seal in the perfume, helping the pot-pourri to fully absorb scent. Place the pot-pourri mix in the container and lay the trimmings on top so that they too absorb scent. Seal and leave to mature for at least two weeks, or anything up to six weeks.

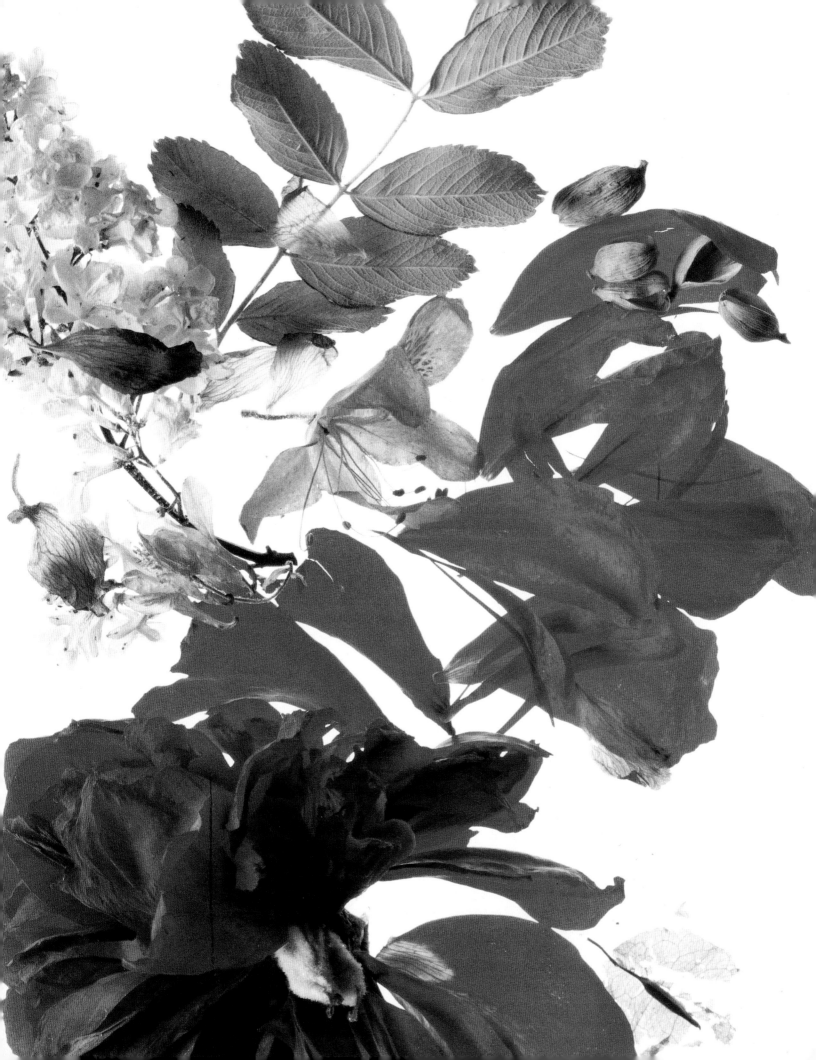

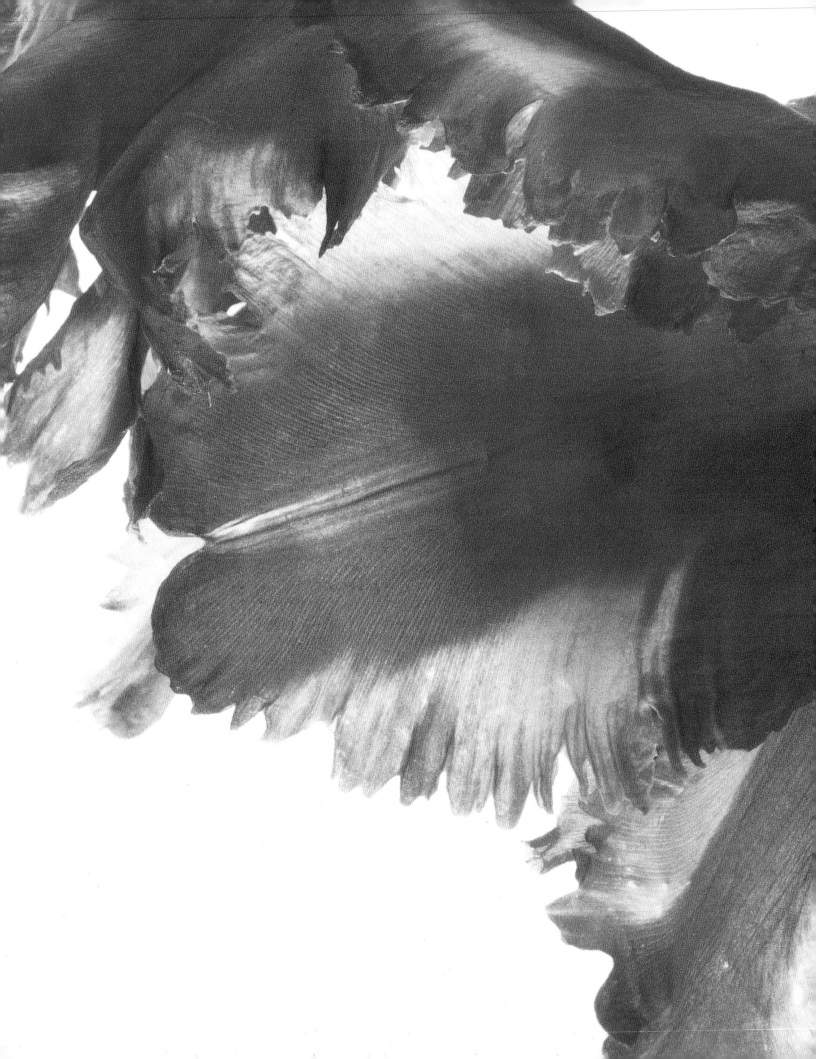

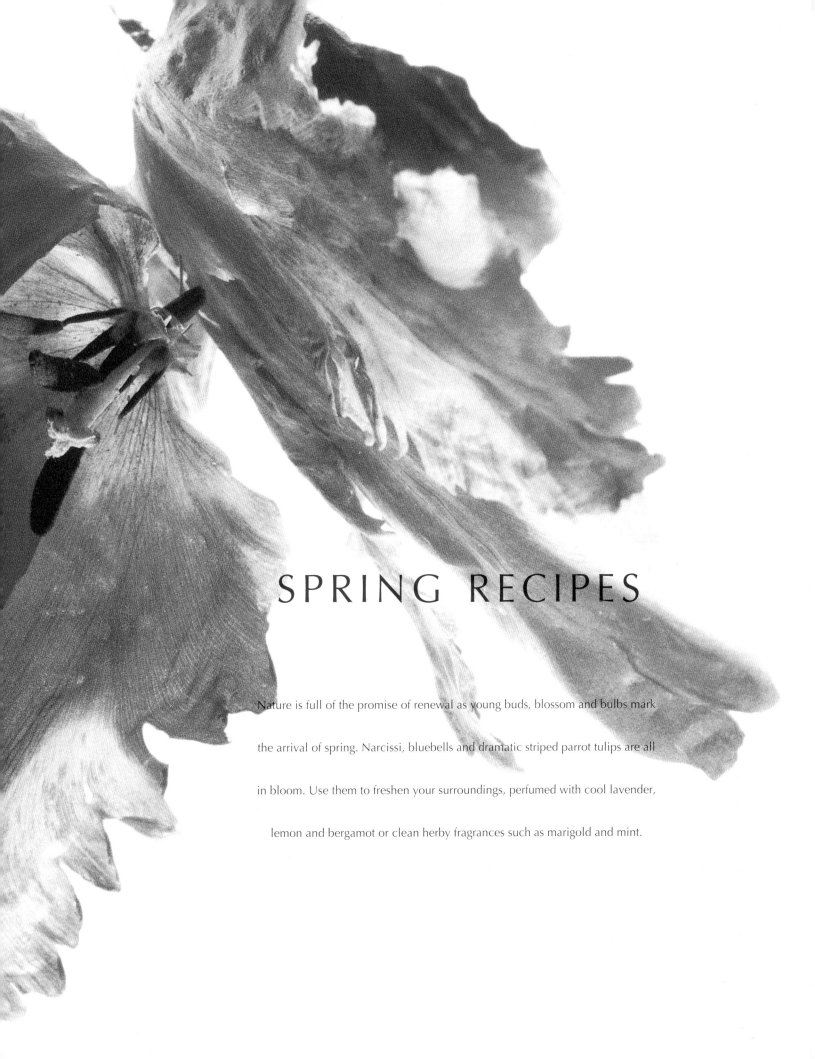

SPRING RECIPES

Nature is full of the promise of renewal as young buds, blossom and bulbs mark

the arrival of spring. Narcissi, bluebells and dramatic striped parrot tulips are all

in bloom. Use them to freshen your surroundings, perfumed with cool lavender,

lemon and bergamot or clean herby fragrances such as marigold and mint.

Melissa and Primavera Pot-Pourris

Melissa is commonly called lemon balm, which was once a staple of cottage gardens and known as "cottager's tea." The herb is valued for its restorative and invigorating qualities. This mix, with its fresh lemon and bergamot fragrance and clean top notes of lavender and eucalyptus, is beneficial for our well-being. Like a ray of spring sunshine, it is full of yellow flowers: there are double daffodils, large African marigolds, sprays of mimosa and Achillea filipendulina 'Goldplate,' all air dried and topped with decorative dried lemon slices.

Primavera is a tribute to Botticelli's famous painting of Primavera and her maidens, decked with flowers. The mix is topped with desiccant-dried spring flowers including huge parrot tulips, pale daffodils, ranunculus and polyanthus, combined with hyacinths, mimosa, cypress tips and ivy leaves to make a flower arrangement in a bowl. It is perfumed with a touch of citrus on a mossy base of galbanum and cypress.

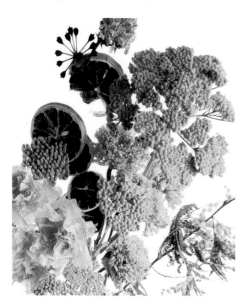

MELISSA

Beloved of bees, melissa takes its name from the Greek word for bee and has a unique honeyed, lemon herbal scent. Since true melissa oil is too expensive to use in pot-pourris, this cheerful blend of golden-yellow flowers is perfumed with a refreshing and invigorating citrus, herby scent of lemon, bergamot and lavender, with a zest of lemon grass and hint of eucalyptus.

THE INGREDIENTS
THE BASE PLANTS
8oz mix of dried yellow
flowers: narcissi, sunflower petals etc
3oz dried eucalyptus leaves
3oz dried lemon peel
2oz dried lemon balm (melissa) or
lemon verbena
THE OILS
100 drops lemon
80 drops bergamot
60 drops lavender
40 drops lemon grass
20 drops eucalyptus
THE POWDERS
1oz orris root
THE CARRIER MATERIALS
2oz coriander seeds
½oz cardamom seeds
1oz senna pods
THE TRIMMINGS
Yellow African marigolds
Achillea filipendulina 'Goldplate'
Double golden-yellow daffodils
Mimosa sprays
Ivy berries
(All the above are air dried)
Lemon slices (radiator dried)

PRIMAVERA

Dried daffodils and mosses are scented with cypress and galbanum, palmarosa and lily-of-the-valley and sharpened with grapefruit, an important part of this springtime blend.

THE INGREDIENTS
THE BASE PLANTS
8oz mix of dried spring flowers:
daffodils, narcissi, tulips, ranunculus etc
3oz clean, dried moss
3oz dried cypress tips, or other evergreen (hedge trimmings are ideal)
2oz small, green, dried ivy leaves
THE OILS
100 drops cypress
80 drops palmarosa
60 drops grapefruit
40 drops galbanum
20 drops lily-of-the-valley (synthetic)
THE POWDERS
1oz orris root
½oz gum benzoin
THE CARRIER MATERIALS
2oz green cardamom husks, or small,
dried green leaves such as myrtle
THE TRIMMINGS
Whole red and yellow parrot tulips
Pale yellow trumpet daffodils
Orange, red and yellow wallflowers
White double-flowered zinnias
Yellow and red polyanthus
White clematis
Mimosa
Kerria japonica (Bachelor's buttons)
Ranunculus
Blue hyacinths
(All the above are silica dried)
Cypress tips and ivy leaves (air dried)

ABOVE LEFT: The trimmings for the Melissa pot-pourri. OPPOSITE: Top dressing for the Primavera pot-pourri.

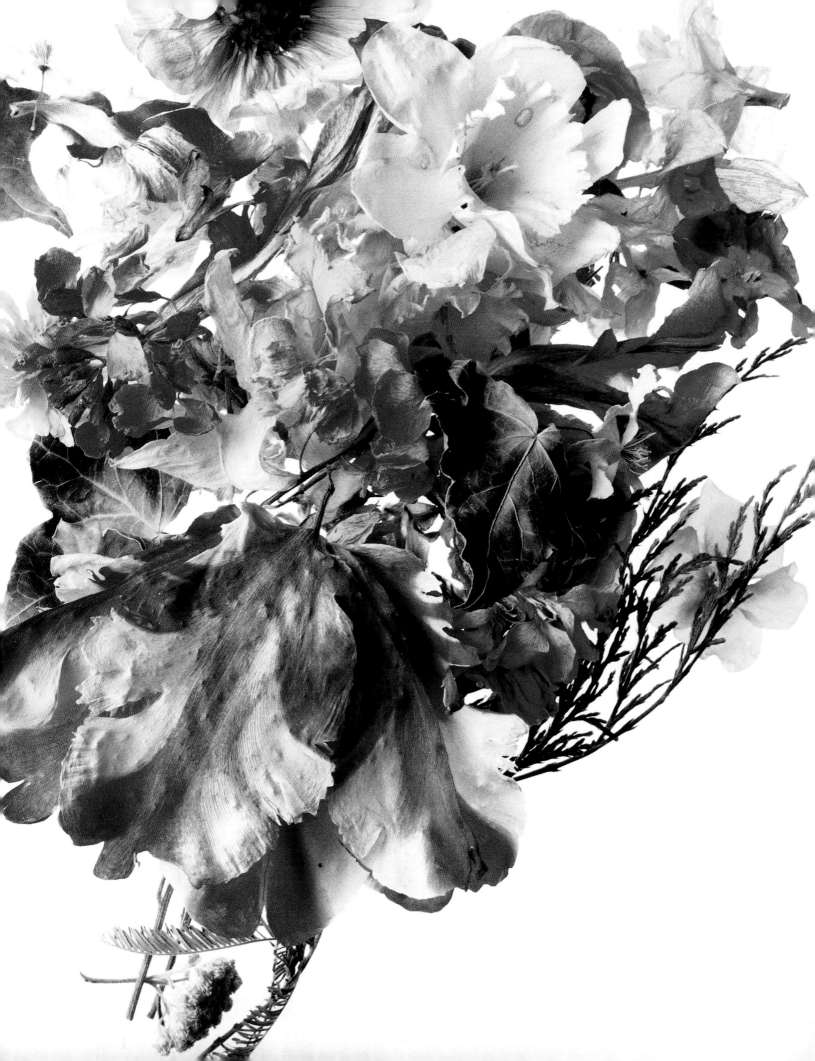

Marigold-and-Mint and Potager Pot-Pourris

Some years ago I came up with the idea of making a pot-pourri to use in dining rooms and kitchens. While spicy scents blend quite happily with food smells, a rich floral aroma would be much less pleasant. In answer to this I produced Marigold-and-Mint, a blend of orange-gold flowers with a fruity, herbal scent of orange and lemon, lavender, marjoram and thyme.

My vegetable pot-pourri, Potager, is named in honor of the ornamental kitchen gardens which are currently undergoing a revival. Vegetables are often beautiful plants, and should not be banished to some untidy patch hidden away from the rest of the garden. Many leaf vegetables dry well (though you should avoid cabbage, which develops a nasty smell), and the curly kale which I have used here is not only decorative but also absorbs fragrance well. Dried peppers and chilis, sliced kiwi fruit and whole lemons add the finishing touches to this spicy, herbal pot-pourri.

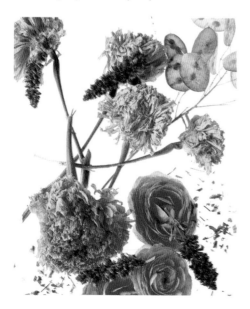

MARIGOLD-AND-MINT

This golden, orangey-yellow pot-pourri has a refreshing citrus, herby scent which makes it particularly suitable for use in kitchens and dining rooms. The marigolds or *calendula* are infused with an aroma I adapted from old recipes for stewing herbs. The green honesty seedheads and scented purple agastache provide some color contrast.

THE INGREDIENTS

THE BASE PLANTS

6oz dried calendula

4oz dried sunflower petals or other yellow flowers

3oz dried lavender flowers, removed from the stem

2 oz dried eucalyptus leaves

1oz whole dried mint leaves

THE OILS

100 drops orange

60 drops lemon

60 drops bergamot

60 drops lavender

20 drops spearmint

THE POWDERS

1 oz orris root

THE CARRIER MATERIALS

1oz coriander seeds

1oz dried mint

½oz dried marjoram

½oz dried thyme

THE TRIMMINGS

Orange African marigolds or calendulas

Physalis (Chinese lanterns)

Purple agastache sprigs

Green honesty seedhead sprays

(All the above are air dried)

Orange ranunculus (silica dried)

POTAGER

This "vegetable" pot-pourri is trimmed with freeze-dried pimento and kiwi fruit, together with chillies, kale and dried lemons. Star anise gives spice to the blend, while the tiny black cardamom seeds are very pungent and help to carry the scent throughout the blend.

THE INGREDIENTS

THE BASE PLANTS

6oz dried calendulas or other golden-yellow flowers

4oz dried sunflower petals or other golden-yellow flowers

3oz dried lavender flowers

2oz whole dried bay leaves

1oz whole dried mint leaves

THE OILS

80 drops orange

80 drops lemon

80 drops bergamot

20 drops basil

20 drops clary sage

10 drops thyme

THE POWDERS

½oz gum benzoin

1oz orris root

THE CARRIER MATERIALS

2oz coriander seeds

1oz dried mixed herbs

1oz cardamom pods or husks

THE TRIMMINGS

Curly kale

Whole chilis

Apple rings and star anise

Whole lemon

(All the above are air dried)

Pimento halves (radiator dried)

Kiwi fruit slices

ABOVE LEFT: *The trimmings for the Marigold-and-Mint pot-pourri.* OPPOSITE: *Plant material for top dressing the Potager pot-pourri.*

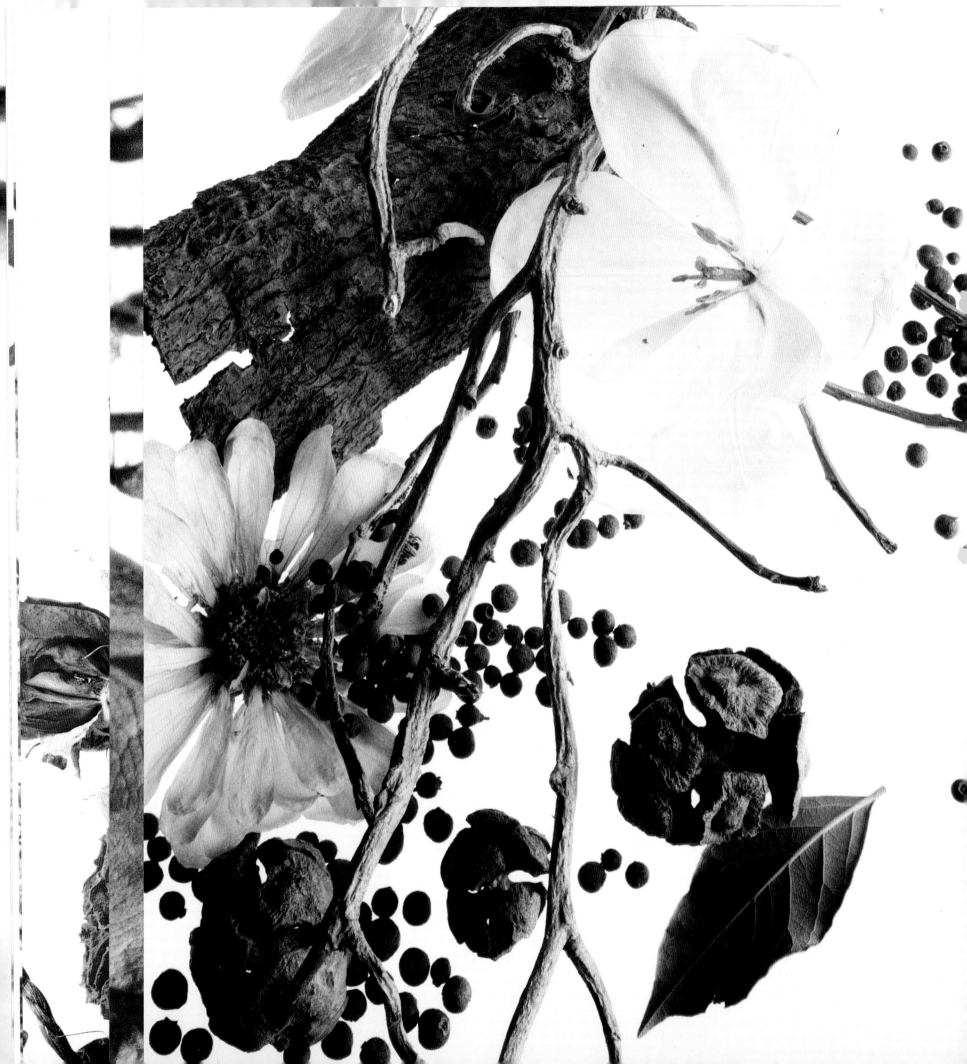

Coromandel and Avalon Pot-Pourris

These two pot-pourris reflect the last golden days of summer. Coromandel ware was highly fashionable in England during the 17th century when cabinets and huge screens were imported to Europe from the Malay peninsula. The plant materials in this mix are woody and exotic, to reflect the inlaid lacquer work after which the pot-pourri is named. This mix includes lemon, clove and rose, but in different proportions to Avalon. With the deep, woody note of Texas cedarwood these fragrances give a richer scent with a gentle citrus top note and a heart of rose and clove.

In Arthurian legend, Avalon was an orchard, "a place where apples grow," and the final resting place of King Arthur. The Avalon mix is trimmed with dried orchard fruits. Both apples and pears are often cooked with lemon and cloves, and these two important aromatics, blended with a synthesized apple fragrance, create a spicy apple scent on a cedarwood base, with just a hint of rose.

COROMANDEL

The two cedarwood oils used in this pair of recipes are very different in character and give each pot-pourri its unique fragrance. The Texas cedarwood oil in Coromandel is deeper and richer than the Virginian cedar which lends its fresh note to the apple scent of Avalon. The ingredients needed for a mix like Coromandel are fairly heavy. It is not always easy to achieve a balance between weight and bulk, but some ingredients, like land lotus petals, appear solid but actually weigh very little. If the trimmings are hard to obtain, substitute plant materials with a carved, woody quality. Powders are omitted from this recipe as they would detract from the shiny "lacquered" feel of the ingredients.

THE INGREDIENTS

THE BASE PLANTS

4oz dried cotton husk flowers

4oz dried land lotus petals

3oz dried coco flowers

5oz mix of small cones

THE OILS

120 drops Texas cedarwood

80 drops rose-scented (synthetic)

80 drops lemon

20 drops clove bud

THE CARRIER MATERIALS

3oz broken cassia bark

1oz coriander seeds

THE TRIMMINGS

Swirled platyspermum cones

Cluster gums (mace)

Palm mule rings or Rams' heads

Kushi fruit

Brachychiton pods

Aristea sprigs (air dried)

AVALON

Although freeze-dried fruits are available, the dried orchard fruits used to trim this pot-pourri are easily made at home. Choose apples with richly colored skins and do not peel or core them. Simply slice across thinly to show the star-shape of pips in the middle and leave a rim of peel around the edge of the fruit flesh. Slice pears lengthways to keep their typical shape. Lay the fruit on racks to dry in a warm, airy place: near a radiator or a central-heating boiler is ideal.

THE INGREDIENTS

THE BASE PLANTS

6oz mix of dried yellow flowers: roses, sunflowers etc

3oz whole cassia bark

3oz dried rosehips

3oz mix of small cones

1oz dried bay leaves

THE OILS

140 drops apple-scented (synthetic)

80 drops Virginian cedarwood

40 drops clove bud

20 drops lemon grass

20 drops rose-scented (synthetic)

THE POWDERS

1oz orris root

½ level teaspoon clove

THE CARRIER MATERIALS

2oz coriander seeds

1oz chopped dried lemon peel

THE TRIMMINGS

Apple rings (air dried)

Pear slices (air dried)

Green hellebore flowers (air dried)

Small white daisies (air dried)

Yellow roses (silica dried)

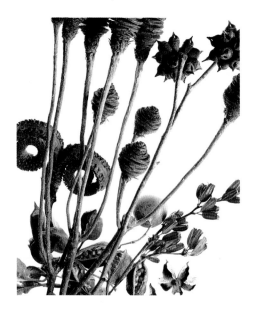

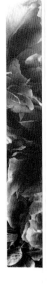

ABOVE LEFT: *Sculpted trimmings for the Coromandel pot-pourri.* OPPOSITE: *Top dressing for the Avalon pot-pourri.*

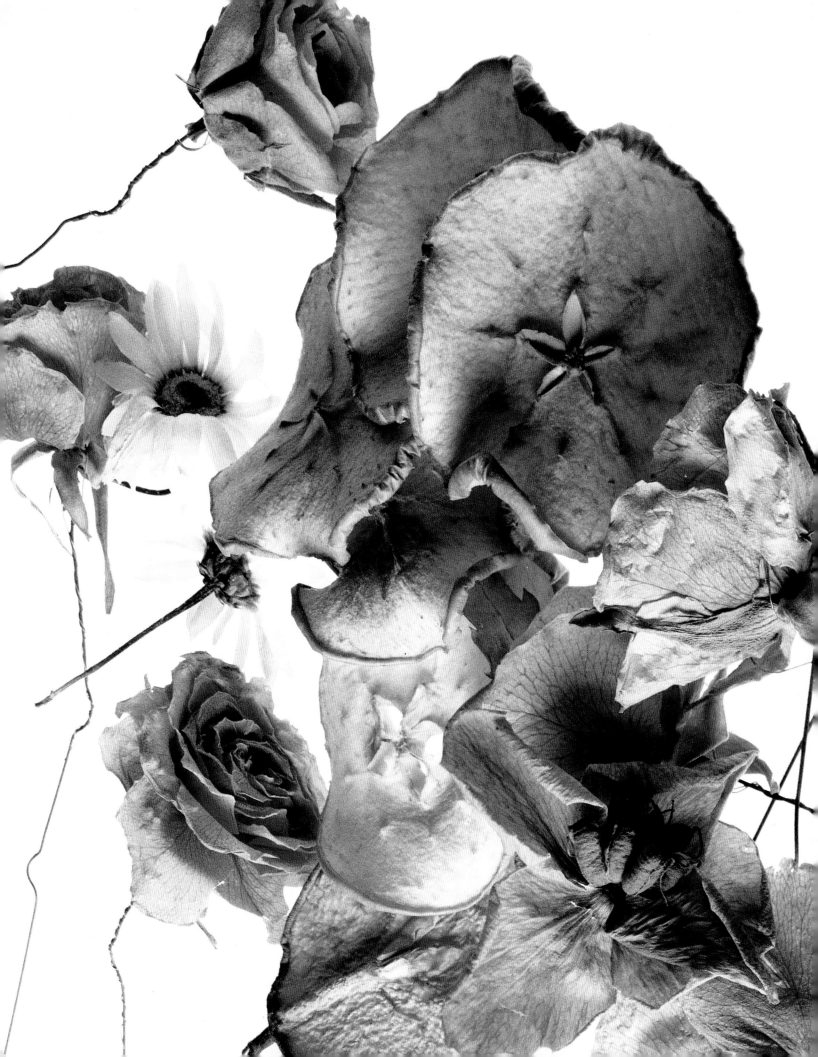

Cyprian and Nut Parchment Pot-Pourris

*W*hen summer has passed and the days start to draw in, we can look for a new fragrance for the home – something warmer than the lavenders and lemons that provided us with cool refreshing scents on the hottest days. Although the flower perfumes of high summer come back into their own in the depths of winter, we are not ready for them just yet. These two recipes were originally created for men, but they are entirely appropriate to the season, and women love them too. Cyprian derives its name from an 18th-century wig powder! It has a resinous, woody base with a touch of spice and a citrus top note.

Nut Parchment came about after I took delivery of some seedpods from the Far East. There were great flat, brown-papery pradu flowers, polished brown seedheads and tissue-paper-thin fiber flowers, which are also seedheads. They constituted a wonderful vehicle to carry a vanilla-based scent with a hint of spice and a fruity top note.

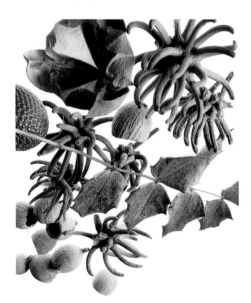

CYPRIAN

During the 18th century when elaborate, towering wigs were fashionable, oakmoss was frequently used as an ingredient in wig powders which, together with powdered orris root and rose petals "served to keep them fragrant and discourage vermin." Here I have used a soft gray-green mix of oakmoss, eucalyptus leaves and senna pods as a plant base to create a subtle pot-pourri with a dry, slightly resinous scent. The senna pods add interest to the mix and are an ideal carrier material for the perfume. Top this neutral blend with interesting seedheads and leaves. There are no powders in the recipe.

THE INGREDIENTS
THE BASE PLANTS
6oz cypress cones or grayish-brown seedheads eg eucalyptus pods
4oz washed, dried, torn oak moss
4oz senna pods
2oz gray-green eucalyptus leaves
THE OILS
100 drops juniper
80 drops bergamot
60 drops cypress
40 drops bois de rose or rosewood
20 drops clary sage
THE CARRIER MATERIALS
2oz senna pods
1oz cardamom husks
1oz chopped calamus root
THE TRIMMINGS
Land lotus petals
Laranja nut
Spider gums
Gum nuts or papri cups
Mahonia japonica leaves (air dried)

NUT PARCHMENT

I have substituted more readily available leaves and pods for the exotic far-eastern plant materials that originally inspired this recipe. I polished some ingredients such as the nuts with the blended oils to intensify the color and add scent to the mix.

THE INGREDIENTS
THE BASE PLANTS
6oz mixed dried pale-colored seed-heads, poppies, liquidambar, sycamore, pradu flowers (if available)
4oz mixed dried fallleaves (try to include sun-bleached varieties)
3oz Douglas fir cones
1oz sun-bleached bells of Ireland
1oz honesty seedpods
THE OILS
120 drops vanilla-scented (synthetic)
80 drops Texas cedarwood
60 drops orange
20 drops cinnamon
20 drops clove
THE POWDERS
1oz powdered orris root
½oz powdered gum benzoin
¼oz ground nutmeg
1 level teaspoon each of ground nutmeg, cinnamon and clove
THE TRIMMINGS
Poppy seedheads (bleached)
Cinnamon quills
Ginko leaves (pressed)
Eucalyptus leaves (bleached)
Walnuts
Sponge mushroom
Honesty seedheads (air dried)
Bell cups

ABOVE LEFT: *The trimmings for the Cyprian pot-pourri.* OPPOSITE: *Plant material to top dress the Nut Parchment pot-pourri.*

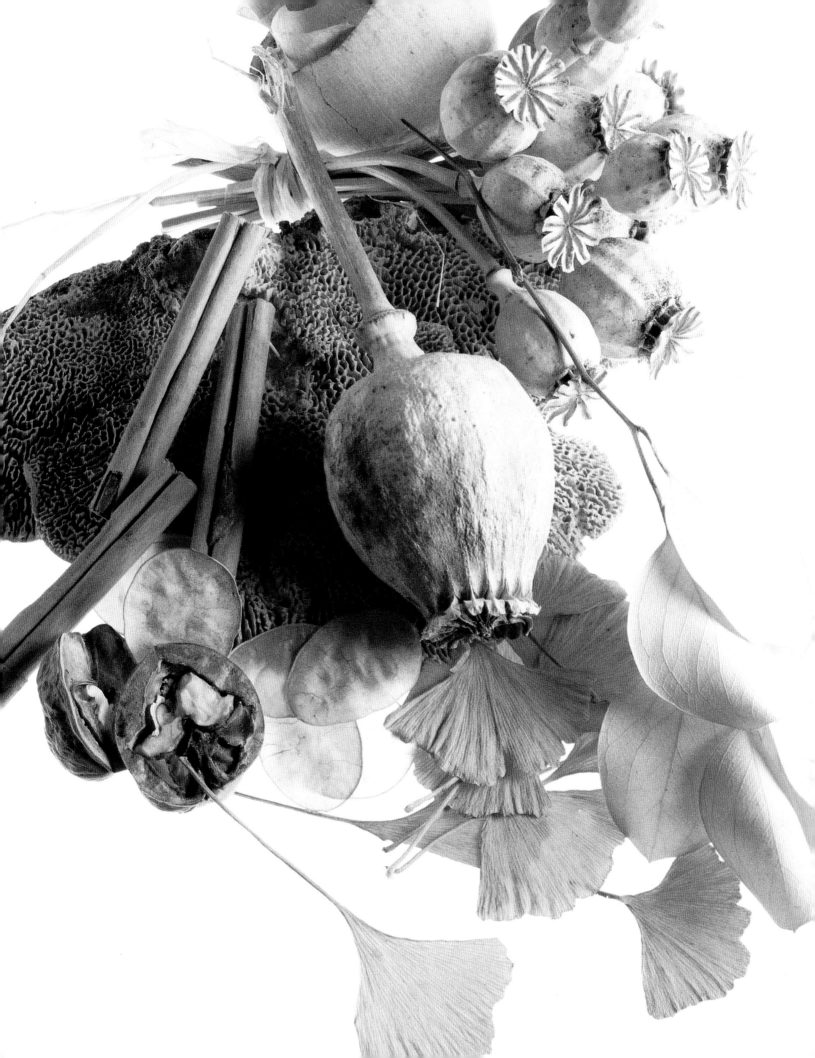

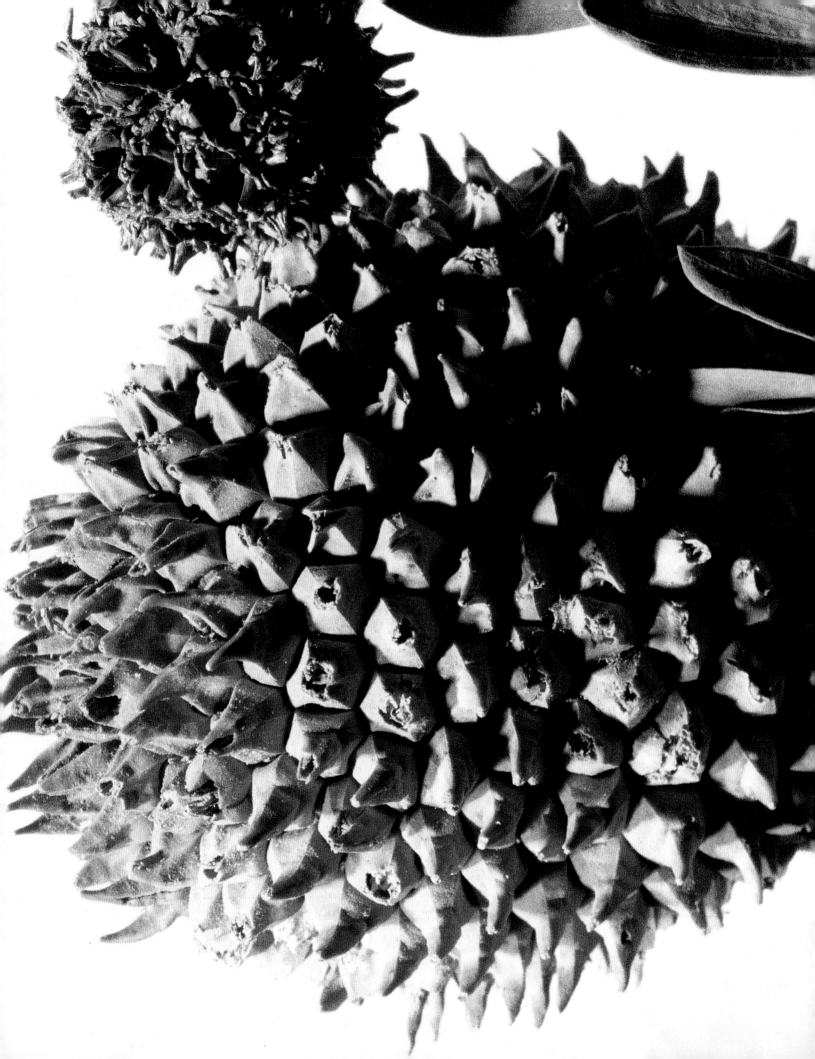

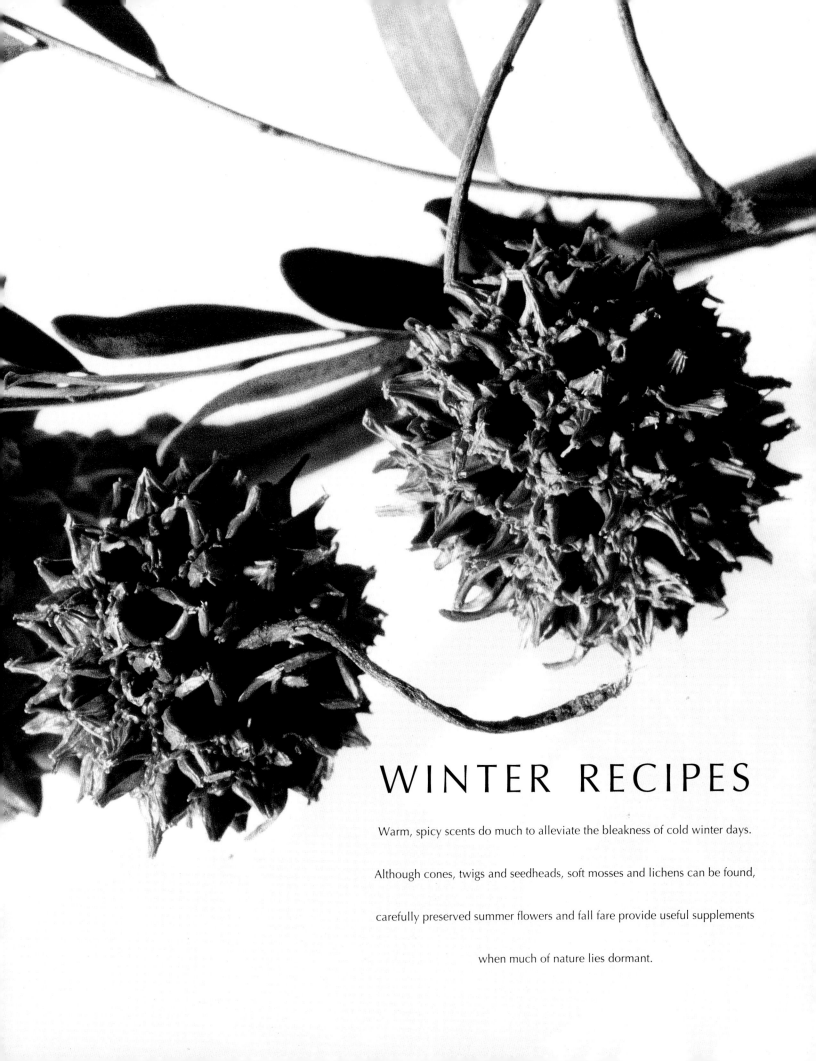

WINTER RECIPES

Warm, spicy scents do much to alleviate the bleakness of cold winter days.

Although cones, twigs and seedheads, soft mosses and lichens can be found,

carefully preserved summer flowers and fall fare provide useful supplements

when much of nature lies dormant.

Zanzibar and Pomander Pot-Pourris

A duo of spicy pot-pourris for the winter season; both feature clove as a major perfume. Zanzibar was inspired by a collection of botanicals. Although they were almost uniform in their soft, grayish-brown hues their forms and textures were diverse. This clove-scented mix is named after the island of Zanzibar where clove seeds were first planted in the late 18th century. Zanzibar and Pemba now produce more than half the world's supply of top-quality cloves.

Pomander suggests the spicy scent of clove oranges. Clove-stuck oranges are the direct descendants of the medieval pommes d'ambre, a name derived from the apple-shaped piece of ambergris from which they were once made. Ambergris, a waxy secretion of the sperm whale, is powerfully fragrant but today it is almost unobtainable. This warm, citrus-scented pot-pourri conjures up the magic of the winter season, a time when bitter Seville oranges are available and spices and aromatics abound in the kitchen.

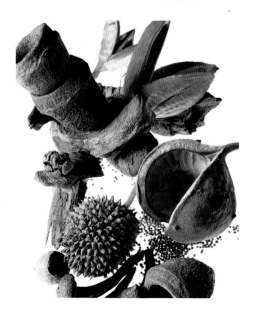

ZANZIBAR

Spicy clove combines with soft vanilla on a base of warm cedarwood, with added zest from the dry note of a touch of black pepper. Pradu flowers are lightweight and absorbent and tone well with the trimmings. Although these flowers are large enough to absorb fragrance by infection, they benefit from being painted with the oil blend. Feel free to substitute materials for those given below.

THE INGREDIENTS
THE BASE PLANTS
7oz dried pradu flowers

5oz whole cassia bar

4oz) cypress cones

THE OILS
100 drops Texas cedarwood

80 drops clove bud

60 drops vanilla

40 drops black pepper

THE POWDERS
¼oz orris root

¼oz gum benzoin

1 level teaspoon clove

1 level teaspoonful nutmeg

(Do not use powders on the trimmings)

THE CARRIER MATERIALS
2oz cassia bark or cinnamon

1oz allspice berries

1oz whole cloves

THE TRIMMINGS
Cup-shaped Brazil nut pods

Lily-like Flora de Madeira

Round, open-sided Buddha nuts

Nail-like preigo

Spiky Jack fruits

Cypress cones

Cardamom, black inner seeds

POMANDER

A delicious spicy, orange-scented pot-pourri with a heady mix of fragrances. It has a rich, warm, aroma that lasts well.

THE INGREDIENTS
THE BASE PLANTS
3oz dried cotton husk flowers

4oz dried orange peel

4oz whole cassia bark

4oz mix of small cones

1oz pradu flowers or brown leaves

THE OILS
100 drops orange

80 drops juniper

60 drops clove bud

40 drops benzoin

20 drops cinnamon

THE POWDERS
¼oz gum benzoin

¼oz orris root

1 level teaspoon clove

1 level teaspoon cinnamon

THE CARRIER MATERIALS
1oz cassia bark, broken small

1oz coriander seeds

1oz whole cloves

1oz allspice

THE TRIMMINGS
Various-sized pomanders (see page 106)

Small bundles of cinnamon quills

Orange peel curls and slices (air dried)

Birch twigs

Whole oranges (radiator dried)

Pradu flowers (air dried)

Cassia bark in large pieces

Liquidambar seedpods (air dried)

Golden mushrooms

Gold-painted cones or nuts (optional)

ABOVE LEFT: *Hard-textured trimmings for the Zanzibar pot-pourri.* OPPOSITE: *Plant material to top dress the Pomander pot-pourri.*

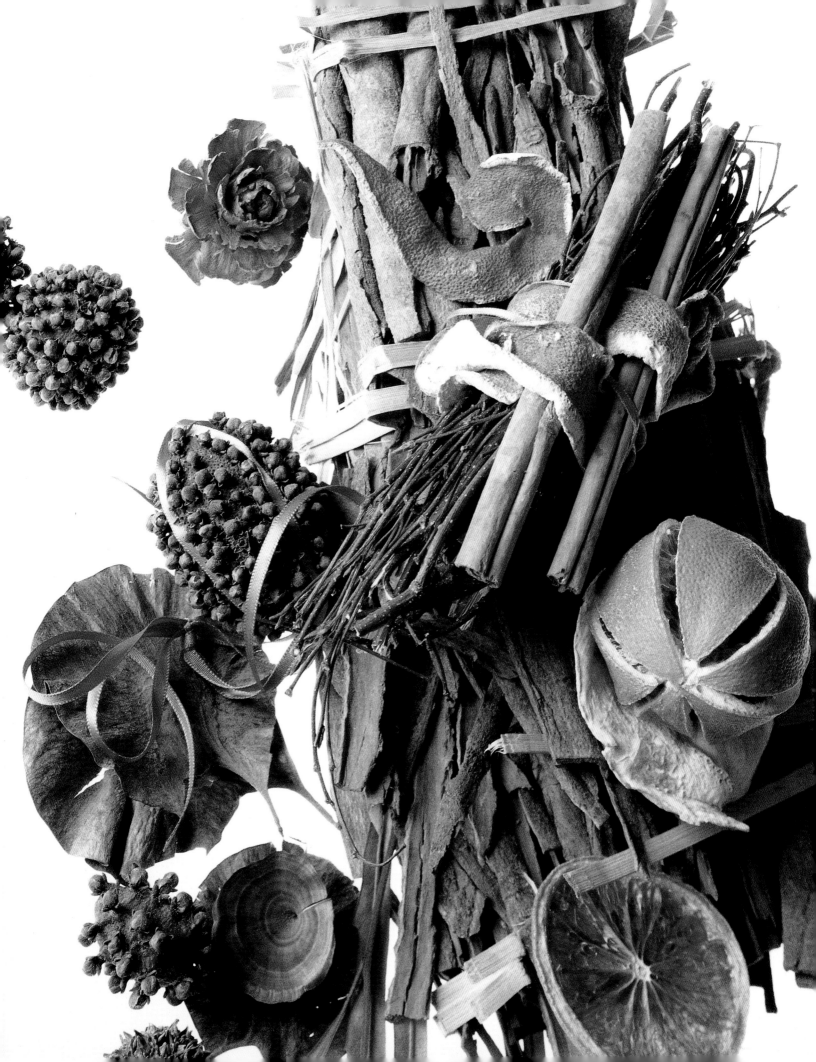

Rosalba and Tudor Rose Pot-Pourris

The name Rosalba comes from Rosa alba, the White Rose of York. This pot-pourri reflects all the fragile beauty of the winter garden. The rose scent is mingled with subtle undertones of cedarwood, juniper and clove. Soft, gray eucalyptus bears its leaves throughout the year and cool gray lichens can be found in winter, along with all kinds of fir cones. The silver brunia and lime-like Bali fruits are imports, but the lambs' tails, lilies and delicate white roses are garden flowers, picked in high summer and preserved for winter use.

The Tudors adopted the rose as the symbol of England. They esteemed above all the damask rose, said to have been brought to England by the crusaders from the gardens of Damascus. The Tudors made sweet bags and pot-pourris from the roses they valued so highly, blended with aromatic spices and gums. This pot-pourri continues this tradition; it is full of red roses and luxuriously scented with sandalwood, frankincense and myrrh.

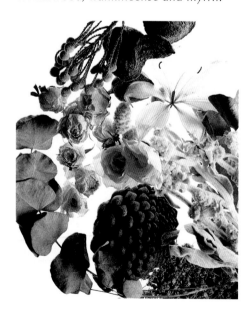

ROSALBA

Virginian cedarwood has long been a classic ingredient of white rose perfume and it is used here to enhance the rose scent and lend a slightly woody note. The black pepper is dry, woody and sweet, while the fresh galbanum gives life to the mosses in the recipe.

THE INGREDIENTS

THE BASE PLANTS

6oz dried eucalyptus leaves

4oz dried oakmoss

2oz dried white rose petals or other small white flowers

4oz grayish cypress cones, larch cones and tiny dark alder cones

THE OILS

100 drops Virginian cedarwood

80 drops juniper

60 drops rose-scented (synthetic)

40 drops black pepper

20 drops galbanum

THE POWDERS

1oz orris root

(Do not use powders on the trimmings)

THE CARRIER MATERIALS

1oz cardamom seeds or husks

1oz juniper berries

1oz whole cloves

THE TRIMMINGS

Eucalyptus sprays (air dried)

Silver-gray lichen moss

White roses (air dried)

White open roses (silica dried)

White lilies (silica dried)

Lambs' ears (air dried)

Silver brunia sprays

Bali fruit husks

A large, heavy grayish-brown cone

TUDOR ROSE

Choose orangey-scarlet roses for drying to make this traditional pot-pourri. Note that flowers always darken when they dry so deep-colored red roses will dry almost black. Trim the mix with red peonies and open red roses (dried in silica gel to preserve their full size and form), sprays of myrtle and fronds of velvety green moss, with perhaps a few small gold leaves, cones or nuts.

THE INGREDIENTS

THE BASE PLANTS

10oz dried red roses

3oz dried velvety moss

2oz tiny alder or larch cones

1oz dried rose leaves

THE OILS

120 drops rose-scented (synthetic)

80 drops sandalwood

40 drops frankincense

40 drops myrrh

20 drops black pepper

THE POWDERS

¼oz orris root

¼oz gum benzoin

(Do not use powder if the pot-pourri is in a glass container; add 10 drops of liquid gum benzoin to the oils)

THE CARRIER MATERIALS

2oz allspice berries

1oz whole cloves

1 cinnamon stick, broken small

THE TRIMMINGS

Whole red peonies (silica dried)

Whole red roses (silica dried)

Tiny red roses on stems (air dried)

Sprays of myrtle leaves (air dried)

Fronds of velvety moss (dry and clean)

ABOVE LEFT: *Trimmings for the Rosalba pot-pourri.* OPPOSITE: *Plant material to top dress the Tudor Rose pot-pourri.*

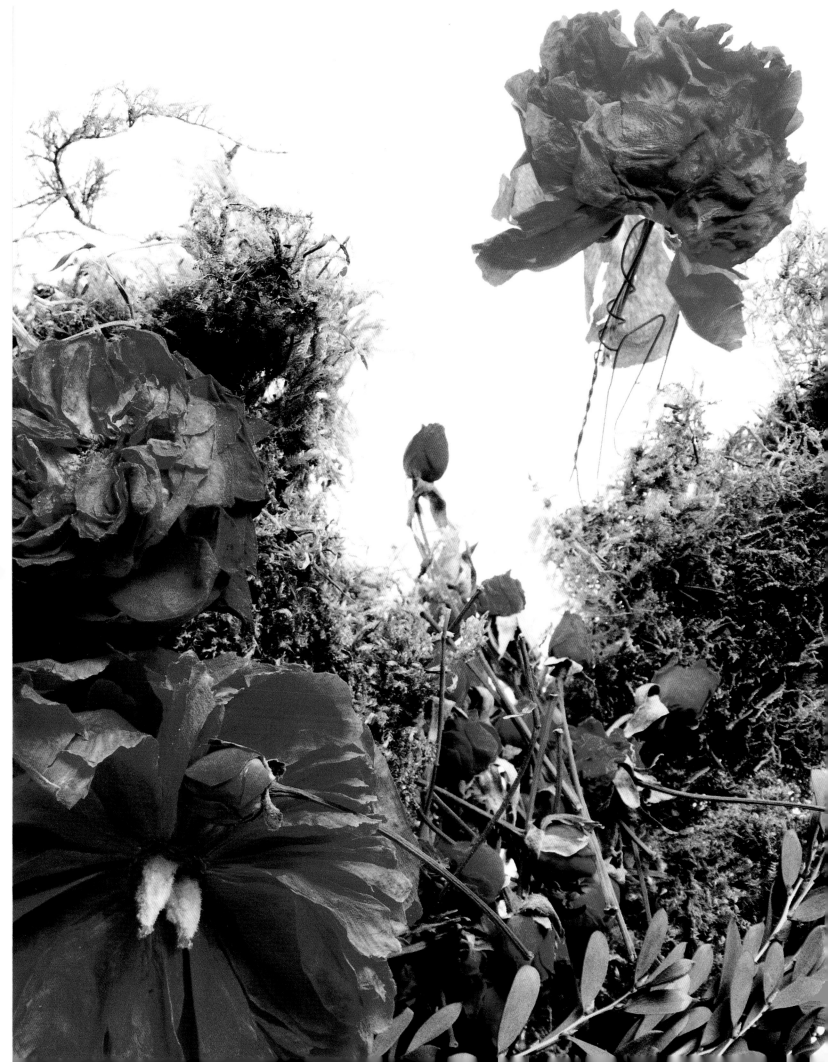

Lavender Bag and Moth Mouse

*F*ragrant bags and sachets are popular
for giving as gifts to add a light floral
scent to clothes, and the bags shown here
are very easy to make.

MATERIALS

16in square cotton fabric

(for the lavender bag)

Elastic band

Ribbon ½in wide

10in square crisp cotton fabric

(for the mouse)

Sewing thread

EQUIPMENT

Pair of compasses

Pins and sewing needle

Scissors and pinking scissors

LAVENDER-BAG MIX

DRIED HERBS

8 cups lavender

1 cup peppermint

1 cup rosemary, rubbed

SPICES

A few whole cloves

MOTH MOUSE MIX

DRIED HERBS

Marjoram

Lavender

Mint

Rosemary

Rue

Southernwood

Sweet woodruff

Tansy

Thyme

SPICES

Cloves, powdered

*A cupful of each of the above mixed
together will yield ten mice. For one
mouse use a tablespoon as the measure*

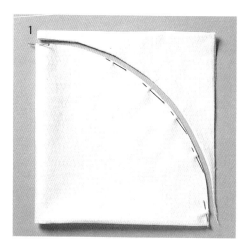

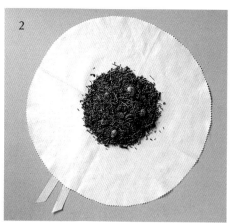

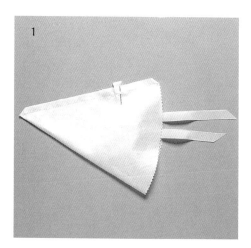

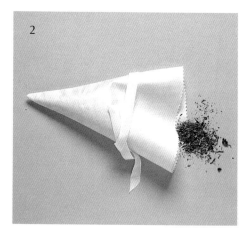

1. Fold the square of cotton fabric exactly into four and press with a cool iron. From the corner where all the folds meet, measure a radius of 8in using the compasses and mark the edge of the quarter circle with pins. Follow the line of pins to cut out and then open out the fabric into a complete circle. (As an alternative, you can use a round plate as a template to cut out a pattern; then pin this to the fabric and cut out the circle.)

2. With the pinking scissors, pink all around the circumference of the circle. Prepare the filling by mixing all the ingredients in a bowl. Lay the fabric on a flat surface and put a cupful of the lavender-bag mix in the middle. Gather up the edges, bunch them together and secure with an elastic band. Finally, tie the neck of the bag with a length of ribbon.

1. Using the compasses, draw out a quarter circle with a 10in radius on the cotton square. Cut out. Pink the rounded edge. Fold into a cone shape with the right sides together. Cut a piece of ribbon 18in long. Angle off each end with a snip. Fold the ribbon in half and pin the fold to the straight edge of the fabric cone, 2in below the pinked edge, with the cut ends of the ribbon inside the cone. Sew a seam ½in in along the straight edge, catching the ribbon fold within the seam. Angle off the seam allowance at each end of the seam.

2. Turn the whole cone right side out and fill it to the level of the ribbon with the mix. Bunch up the open pinked edges and close them by tying the ribbon "tail" in a bow. The finished bag and mouse are shown opposite.

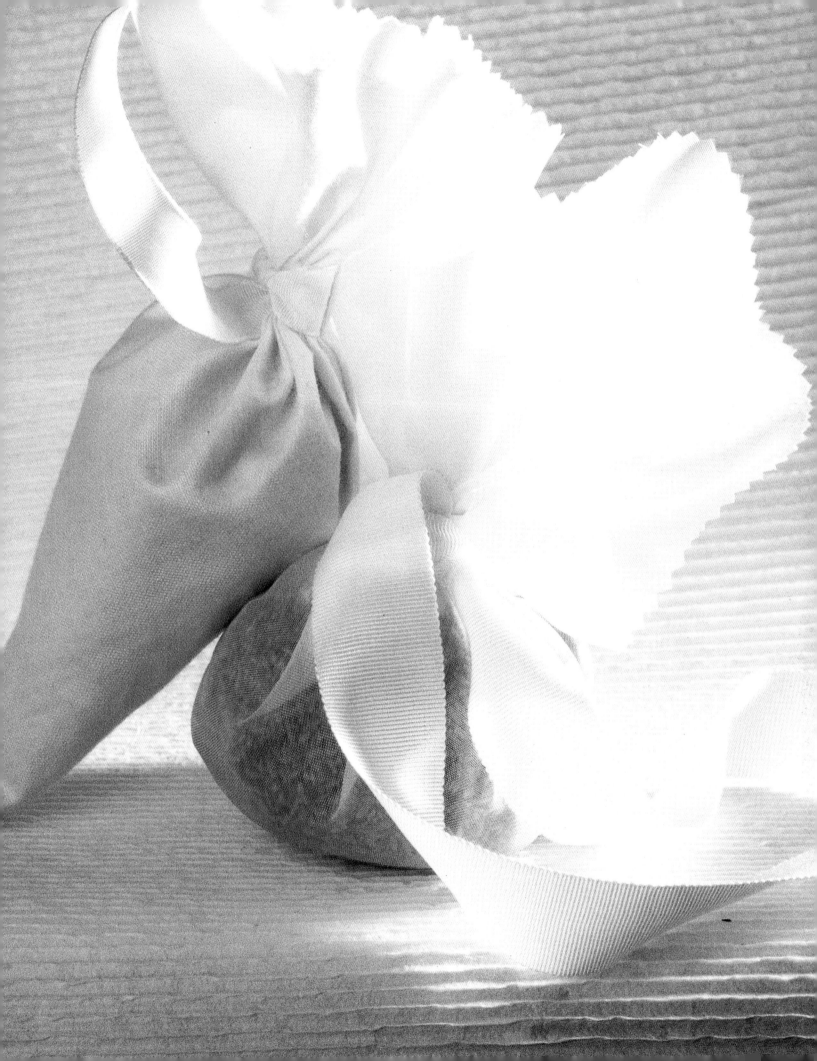

Scented Pillows

*F*ragrant pillows and cushions will help even confirmed insomniacs to enjoy a good night's sleep. I make my scented pillows in two stages. The first involves constructing an inner pad which contains the scented pot-pourri. Then I make an outer casing which I trim with pretty bows. You can trim the outer casing with lace or any other type of finishing to match your bedroom decor. Once you have mastered the basic method, you can make pillows in all shapes and sizes out of all kinds of fabrics, plain or patterned, and filled with any of my pot-pourri mixes for use in other rooms at home (see pages 46-89).

MATERIALS

18 x 12in rectangular piece of cotton fabric

Two 17 x 11in rectangular pieces of batting

Strong sewing thread

29 x 10in rectangular piece of cotton fabric

Ribbon (optional)

EQUIPMENT

Mixing bowl

Pins

Pinking scissors

Sewing needle and thread

SCENTED PILLOW MIX

See right for a selection of different scented pillow mixes.

Whichever mix you choose, you should mix all the ingredients together in a bowl and then set the mixture aside in order to mature for a few days. For best results, seal the mixture inside a poultry roasting bag or in an airtight jar

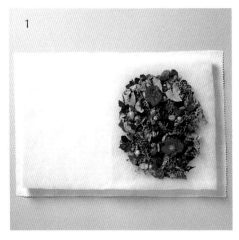

1. First make the scented pad that will go inside the pillow casing. The pad made of batting bulks out the pillow and holds the scented ingredients. Start by pinking all four edges of the 18 x 12in rectangular piece of cotton fabric using the pinking scissors. Then place the pinked rectangle of fabric on a flat surface and position the two rectangular pieces of batting centrally on top of it. Sandwich a layer of your chosen pot-pourri mix (from any recipe given on pages 46-89) between the two layers of batting (this is not visible in the picture above). Then, using a spoon, pile the rest of the pot-pourri mix on top of one half *only* of the top layer of batting, as shown in the illustration above.

LAVENDER MIX

DRIED HERBS AND OTHER PLANTS

2 cups dried lavender flowers

$^1/_2$ cup dried "rubbed" peppermint

(For this ingredient, dry peppermint leaves in a warm place and once brittle simply rub them quite firmly between thumb and forefinger until they crumble)

ESSENTIAL OILS

20 drops lavender

5 drops peppermint

5 drops rose geranium

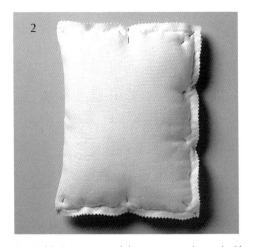

2. Fold the cotton fabric rectangle in half along the two long edges, in order to enclose the batting and the scented, herby mix. Pin the three open edges neatly together and then baste or tack firmly approximately 12mm ($^1/_2$in) in from all three outside edges to catch all the layers together. Do not use a sewing machine to complete the stitching in this step; hand sewing is a much easier way to catch all the layers of fabric together in order to avoid spillage of the scented mix. The illustration above shows the inner scented padding sewn to contain the scent.

ORIENTAL MIX

DRIED HERBS AND OTHER PLANTS

1 cup rose petals and buds

$^1/_2$ cup lavender

$^1/_2$ cup eucalyptus leaves

$^1/_2$ cup oakmoss

$^1/_4$ cup dried rosemary (not powdered)

SPICES

1 cinnamon stick, broken small

6 cloves, whole

ESSENTIAL OILS

10 drops cedarwood

10 drops patchouli

10 drops rose-scented oil (synthetic)

10 drops bergamot

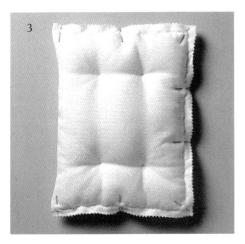

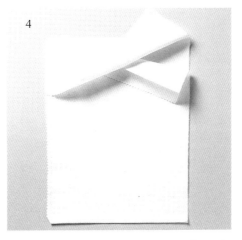

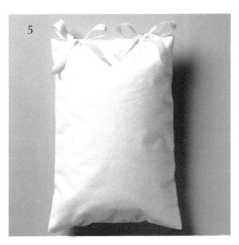

3. If the inner casing containing the scented mix seems slightly insecure then you may feel it necessary to hand stitch four neat catch stitches through all the layers, approximately 2in in from each corner; this will help hold all the layers together. Remove the pins. As an alternative, you may prefer to hand or machine stitch two sides of the inner cotton casing (wrong sides facing) before turning it right side out. Then insert the scented batting. Close the open side of the casing using hand stitches. Whichever method you choose, the above forms the inner padding.

SPICY MIX

DRIED HERBS AND OTHER PLANTS

1¹/₂ cups dried rose petals

¹/₂ cup torn oakmoss

¹/₂ cup sandalwood raspings

ESSENTIAL OILS

10 drops orange

10 drops cedar

5 drops cinnamon

5 drops clove leaf

or

10 drops cedar

10 drops orange

5 drops cinnamon

5 drops clove leaf

4. To make the outer casing or pillow slip take the 29 x 10in rectangular piece of cotton fabric and mark off a 1in turning along one short edge and mark a 4in turning along the opposite short edge of the rectangle; use tailor's chalk or a fabric marker for this purpose. Mark the mid-points of the long edges (these will fall 12 in from each *folded* edge.) Fold the fabric in half lengthways, with right sides facing. Turn the shorter 1in hem over (on to the wrong side of the fabric) and bring the deeper 4in hem over it so that they are both pointing in the same direction, as shown in the picture above. Stitch (by hand or by machine) through all the layers down both long sides on the wrong side of the fabric. Clip the corners just outside the seams to neaten and turn the pillow slip right side out.

SLEEP MIX

DRIED HERBS AND OTHER PLANTS

1 cup lavender

¹/₂ cup chamomile flowers

¹/₂ cup marjoram

¹/₂ cup torn oakmoss

ESSENTIAL OILS

10 drops lavender

10 drops melissa

10 drops petitgrain

5. Having completed step 4 you will now have a hem on one side and a deep flap to hold the pillow in on the other – this is the front. For a final embellishment, cut four equal lengths of ribbon, each one about 8in long. As an alternative (and this is what I did here) you can cut four long narrow strips of matching cotton fabric to the same lengths. Pink the edges of the strips for decorative effect. Make a small fold, about ¼in at one end of each narrow strip. Mark four points (two equally spaced on either side of the opening of the outer casing) with a pin. Hand sew the folded end of each strip of fabric or length of ribbon to these four points. Press the pillow slip and insert the inner casing. Tie the ribbons into two bows to close the mouth of the outer casing.

If you would like to make a so-called "Oxford" pillow casing which has an extended flap, then you should allow an extra 1in of fabric all around. Make up as before and then topstitch 1in in from the edge of the long flap, stopping 1in away from the edges. Carefully pick up the line of sewing and topstitch all around the rest of the casing 1in in from the edge.

A variety of scented pillows in natural shades is shown overleaf.

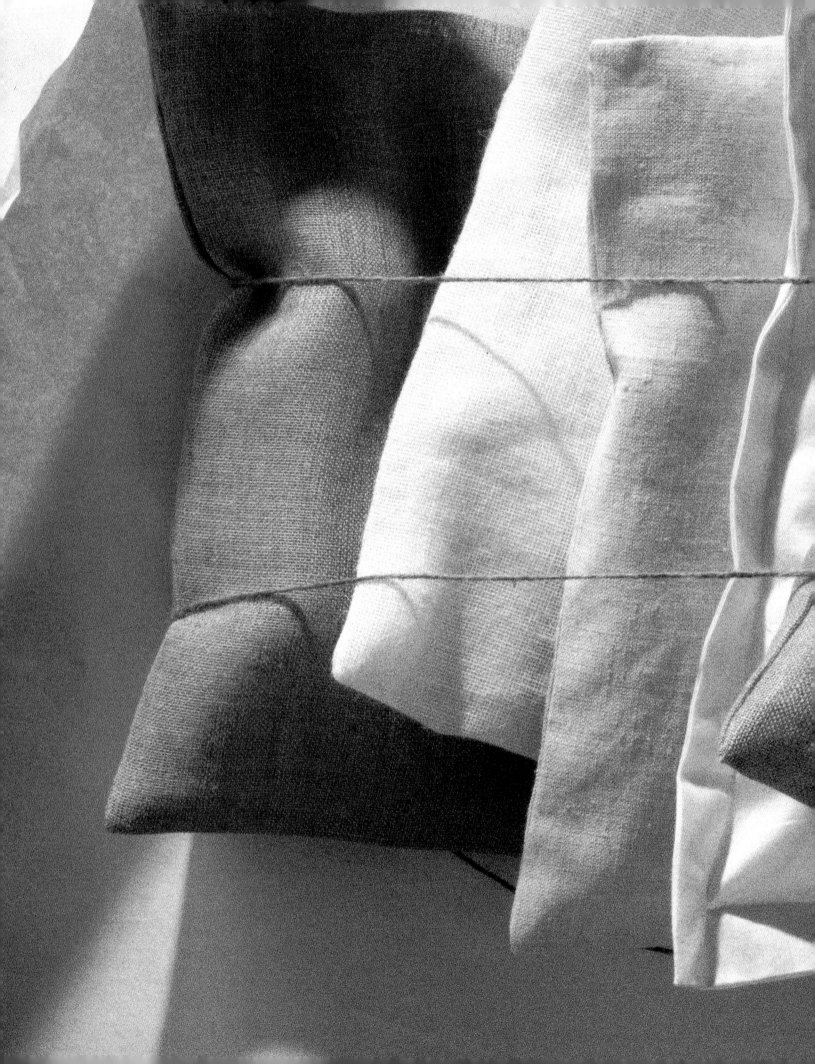

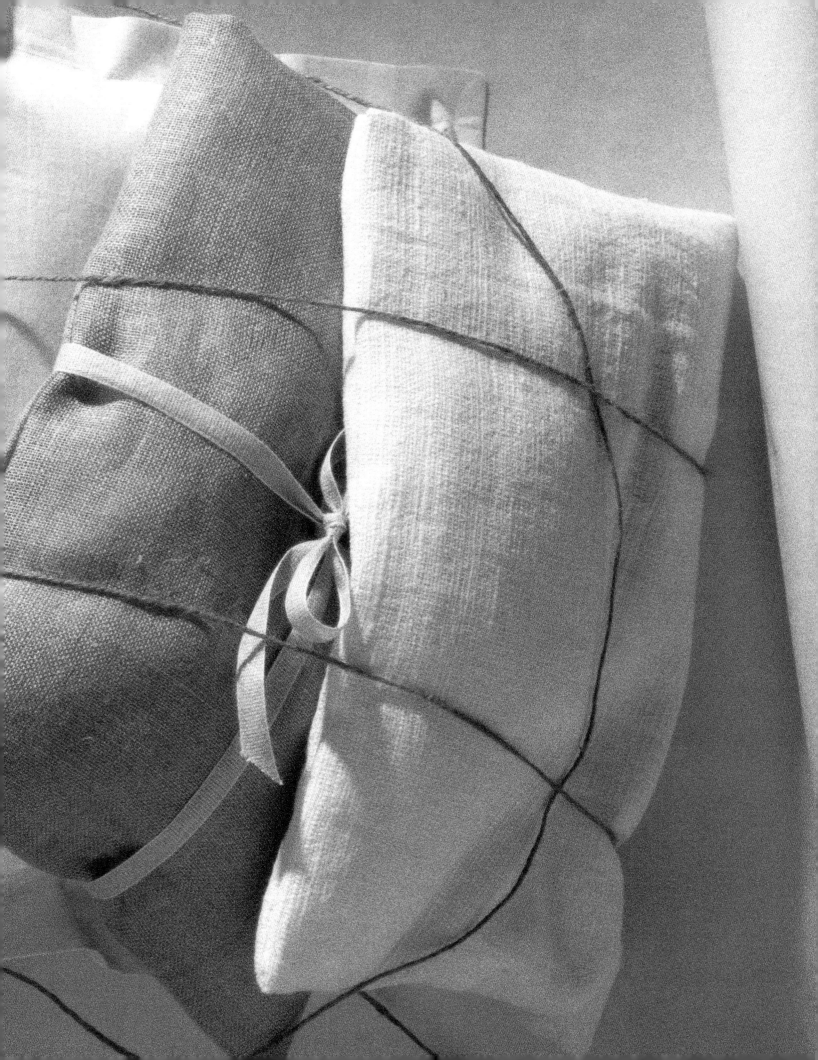

Drawer Liners

Scented papers are perfect for lining drawers to add a subtle fragrance to clothes, handkerchiefs and bed linen. Paper will absorb scent readily, but for our purpose it must be perfumed by "infection," as direct application of the oil to the paper will leave ugly marks and might stain the contents of the drawer. The sachet used here to scent the paper is based on the peau d'Espagne sachets so popular during the 19th century and it has also been used to create the scented writing papers (see page 108). I used a linen scrim to make the sachet, but close-woven fabrics such as cotton are easier to handle and need no interlining.

MATERIALS

26 x 9in fine linen scrim

11 x 14in batting

11 x 14in close-woven fabric or non-woven interlining

Sewing thread

Narrow ribbon

EQUIPMENT

Scissors

Sewing needle

Cellophane sheeting, paper bag with waxed lining or poultry roasting bag

SCENTED FILLING MIX

SPICES

2oz powdered orris root

1oz powdered gum benzoin

ESSENTIAL OILS

Rosewood/cedarwood/sandalwood or

Lavender/patchouli/rose or

Bergamot/lavender/lemon grass

Use 30 drops of each of the oils (all are moth repellent.) Mix all the ingredients together in a bowl ready for use

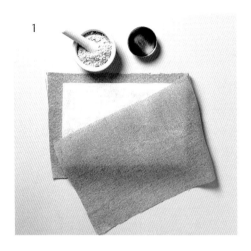

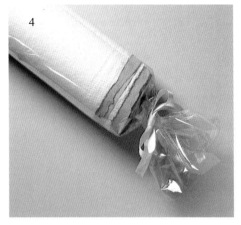

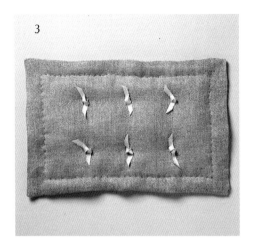

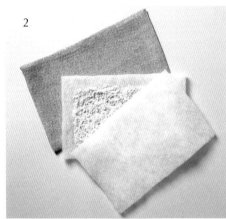

1. Cut the piece of batting into two equal rectangles, each one measuring 11 x 7in. Fold the rectangle of linen scrim in half along the long edge. Prepare the scented filling mix using spices and oils.

2. Machine stitch the linen rectangle about ½in in along both long edges. Clip the corners for a neat finish, turn through and press with an iron. Turn in a 1in hem around the mouth of the linen sachet and press again to give a crisply folded edge.

Cut two rectangles of close-woven fabric or interlining, each one 1 x 7in. Use these to line each piece of batting to retain the filling. With a spoon, scatter a layer of the scented filling onto one layer of batting, with the lining material under it, leaving a 1in margin on all four sides.

3. Place the second batting layer on top of the first to sandwich the scented mix and cover with the lining material. Baste around all four edges of the batting and lining and through all the layers, to hold the scented mix inside. Insert the scented batting into the linen casing and handstitch the mouth of the sachet closed. "Tuft" the sachet with ribbon to hold the layers together; cut short strips of ribbon and hand-stitch them at intervals through all the layers; knot and trim the ends into tufts. Topstitch by hand or machine 1in in from the edges to strengthen.

4. Enclose the linen sachet with your chosen paper in a sealed space using the cellophane sheeting. Keep airtight for several days. The paper will absorb the scent of the mix, ready for use. The sealed paper is shown opposite.

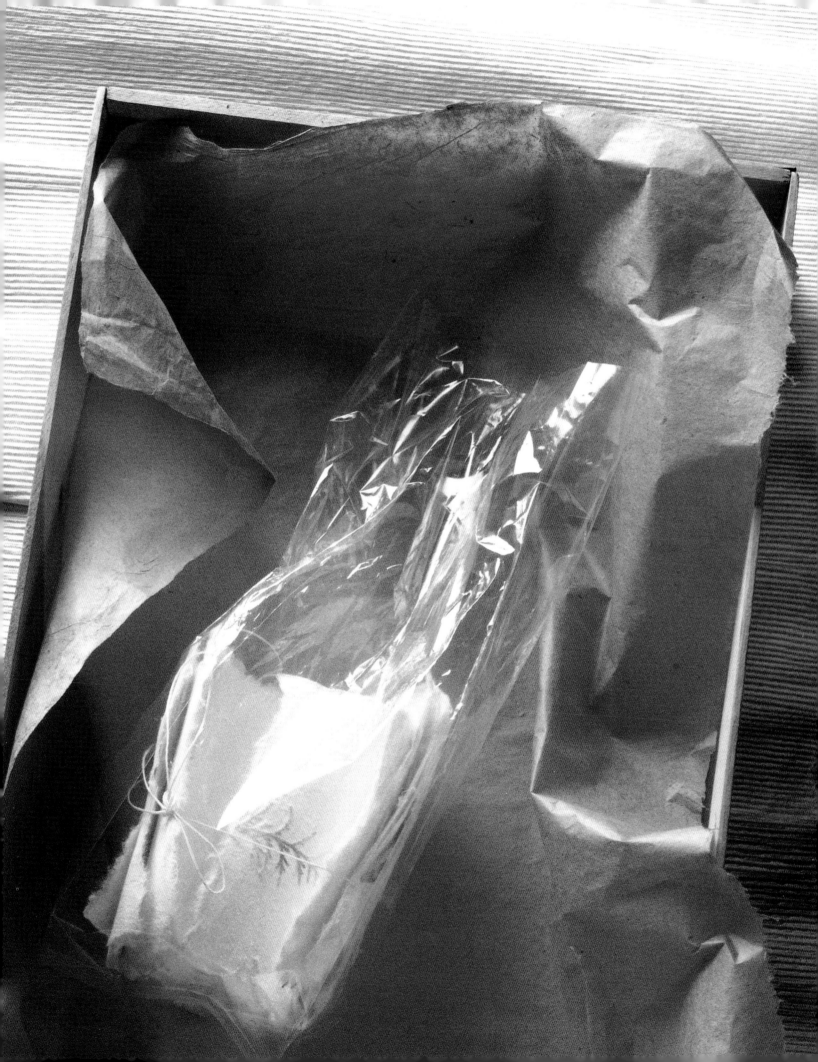

Bath Oils

*A*n aromatic bath can benefit your health and well being. Distribute the oil in the water by hand before you step in. Stay in the bath for a minimum of ten minutes; relax and breathe deeply. Some essential oil molecules will penetrate the skin and others will be inhaled as vapor and diffused from the lungs into the bloodstream and around the entire body. Note that the recipes given for skin types (see immediate right) make up a base or carrier oil blend. To scent the carrier oil blends further refer to the recipes in the far right-hand column. For a full bath use no more than a teaspoon of the oils specified in the recipes.

The carrier oils given in the recipe below will nourish the skin: sweet almond oil is light and good for general use; the avocado and wheatgerm oils are rich in vitamins. Wheatgerm in particular is rich in vitamin E and acts as a natural antioxidant to prevent rancification of the essential oils. Whichever blend of carrier or base oils you choose, I advise you always to include at least 5 percent of wheatgerm oil in the mix.

EQUIPMENT
Clean, empty glass bottle of 3½fl oz capacity (available from a druggist)
Pipette
Small glass funnel
ESSENTIAL OILS
100 drops rosewood
60 drops orange
40 drops petitgrain
CARRIER OILS
2½fl oz sweet almond
⅓fl oz avocado
100 drops wheatgerm

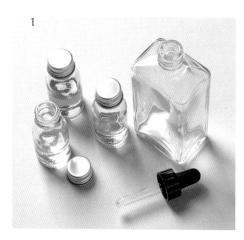

1. The method applies to all the recipes on this page. First assemble your materials. Measure the essential oils into the bottle, using a pipette for accuracy.

CARRIER BATH OIL FOR DRY SKIN
2⅓fl oz apricot kernel
⅓fl oz avocado
⅓fl oz wheatgerm
Apricot kernel oil is beneficial for mature, sensitive and dry skin while the avocado oil is rich in nutrients

CARRIER BATH OIL FOR NORMAL SKIN
1½fl oz sweet almond
1fl oz peach kernel
100 drops wheatgerm
Sweet almond oil is suitable for all skin types; it helps relieve itching, soreness and inflammation. Peach kernel is a light, nourishing oil which keeps the skin smooth and soft

CARRIER BATH OIL FOR OILY SKIN
2½ fl o) hazelnut
⅓fl oz sesame seed
Hazelnut oil is especially good for oily skin as it is slightly astringent. The sesame seed oil prevents rancification

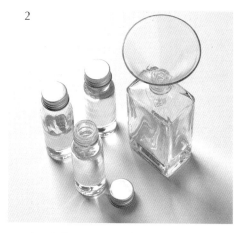

2. Blend the carrier oils in a glass vessel before you add the blend to the essential oils already measured out into the bottle. Replace the cap of the bottle and shake to blend.

MORNING BATH OIL
80 drops lavender
80 drops rosemary
40 drops lemon
3fl oz chosen carrier oil (see left)
A refreshing and invigorating bath to wake up to with a fresh, herbal scent

BEDTIME BATH OIL
80 drops lavender
80 drops rosewood
40 drops chamomile
3fl oz chosen carrier oil (see left)
A magical mixture for a relaxing evening bath as a prelude to a sound night's sleep; the lavender and chamomile are both extremely soothing

ATHLETE'S BATH OIL
80 drops marjoram
80 drops lavender
40 drops rosemary
3fl oz chosen carrier oil (see left)
Helps relieve aches and muscle fatigue

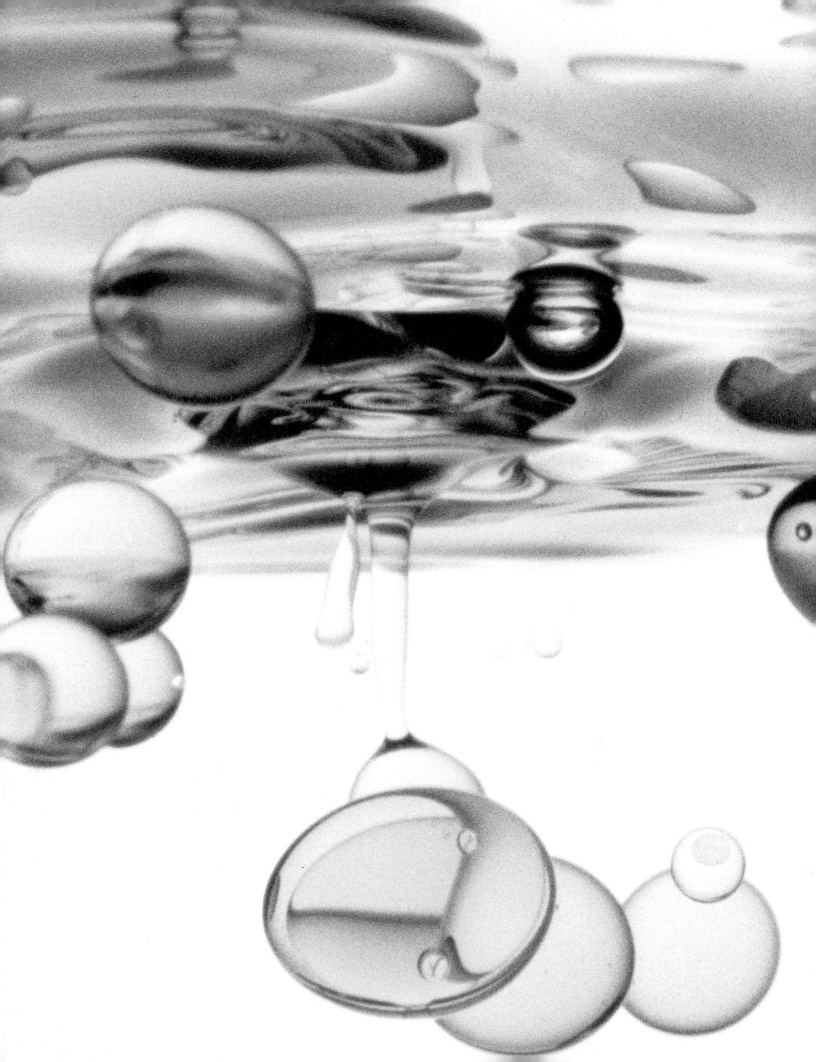

Soap Balls

Scented soap or wash balls in all sorts of fragrances make delightful gifts, or you can pile them high in glass jars or ceramic bowls to use in your own bathroom. It is well worth making your own soap balls in order to incorporate your own favorite treatment oils. As you learn more about the special properties of essential oils you can experiment and begin to produce your own wash balls to relax, invigorate or protect against minor infections. For further information on essential oils and how to combine them, see pages 36-43. As with other recipes using oils, the most accurate method of measurement is to use a pipette.

When making your own soap balls consider using one of the luxury pure essential oils such as rose, sandalwood, jasmine or neroli as a single fragrance. Although these oils are very expensive they are extremely potent and so you only need use very small amounts. Use six to eight drops of these oils to the quantity of soap that is specified in the recipe below. The addition of essential oils slightly alters the original color of the soap. If you wish, you can add a small quantity of food coloring (following the manufacturer's instructions) to color your hand-made soap further.

MATERIALS

5½oz bar of best-quality,
least-scented toilet soap

EQUIPMENT

Mixing bowl

Grater

Bain-marie (double saucepan)

Pestle and mortar

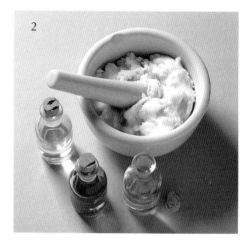

1. Grate the unscented toilet soap into the mixing bowl. The more finely you grate the soap, the smoother the finished texture of the wash ball will be. If you prefer a rough-textured soap then use a coarse grater. An ordinary cheese grater is quite sufficient. Note that the color of the original soap you grate will dictate the color of the finished wash ball. Mix the grated soap with water in the ratio of one part water to two parts soap. Heat over a gentle heat in a bain-marie until the mixture coalesces into a thick paste. This process happens quite slowly. Do not leave the mix unattended on the heat.

LEMON OIL MIX

6 drops lemon

4 drops bergamot

2 drops lemon grass

A fresh and invigorating blend of citrussy oils with cooling scents for a perfect summer soap

OIL MIX TO RELAX AND REVITALIZE

6 drops rosewood

3 drops chamomile

3 drops lavender

Rosewood is a good skin treatment and lavender and chamomile soothe well

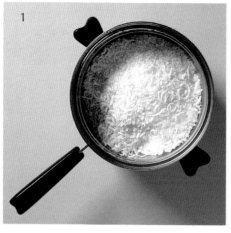

2. Transfer the paste into the mortar and add the chosen combination of essential oils, measuring them accurately with a pipette. See below for effective essential oil mixes. Use the pestle to amalgamate the oils thoroughly with the paste. Do not worry if the paste appears quite wet – this consistency is vital to allow for easy molding of the soap balls. When everything is well mixed, wet your hands, take a small handful of the paste and mold the mixture into neat balls. Leave to cool and set hard. Once hard, the soap balls are ready to use. The finished wash balls are shown opposite.

OIL MIX TO INVIGORATE

6 drops lavender

4 drops geranium

2 drops basil

The clean, herbal scent of basil blended with lavender and geranium provide the perfect "wake-up" soap

OIL MIX TO WARD OFF INFECTION

4 drops tea tree

4 drops lavender

4 drops juniper

A prophylactic blend of oils with antiseptic and antibiotic qualities

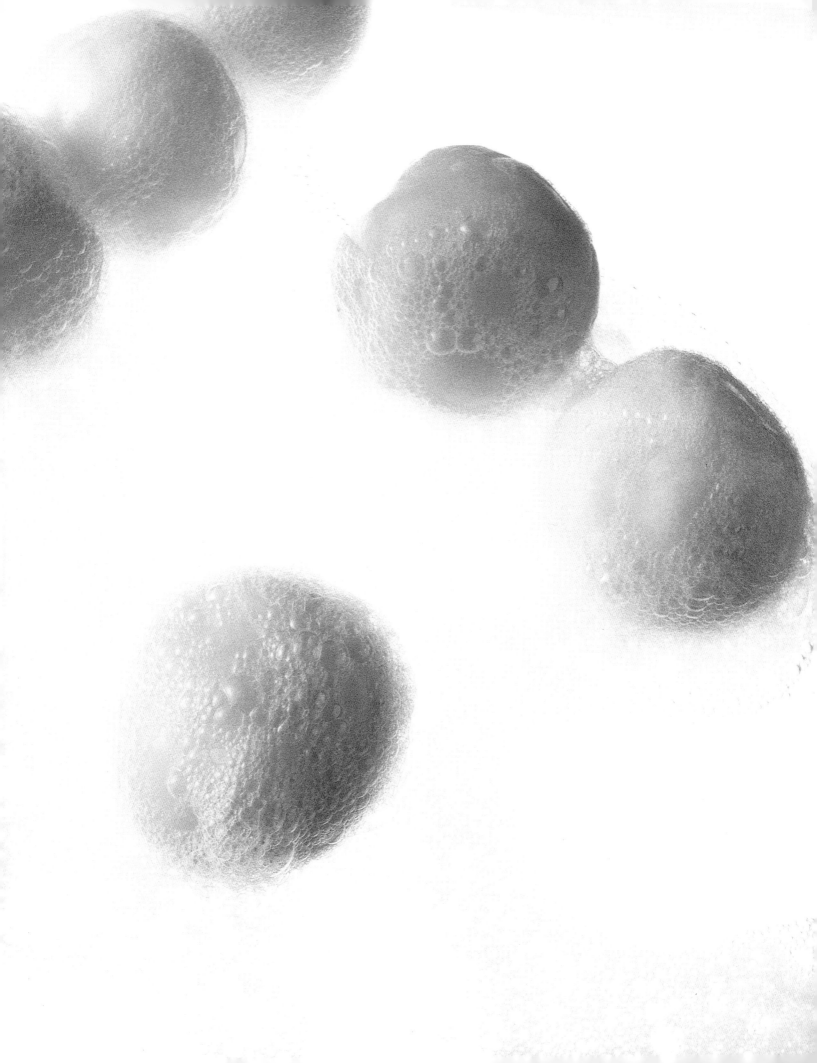

Shell Candle

Shells make charming and unusual containers for scented candles. Make sure that they are absolutely clean and dry and check that there are no holes in the shell before you start. Shell-shaped dishes have been in use for centuries, and these scallop-shell scented candles are appropriate for use on the dinner table to impart a gentle fragrance and light. Keep in mind that the scent of the oil you choose must blend with the food.

MATERIALS

Scallop shell

Miniature wicker ring (to fit shell)

Old candles or candle wax

EQUIPMENT

Glue gun or quick-drying glue

Wick and metal stabilizer (see below)

Small pair of pliers

Metal saucepan

Heat-diffusing mat (optional)

Small ladle

Use a container wick with a lead oxide core; this is safe and burns to a powder. For a 2in diameter candle use a small wick; for a 2-4in diameter candle use a medium wick; use a large wick for a 4-6in diameter candle

Metal stabilizers, also called sustainers, come in two standard sizes: small (shown here) and medium

ESSENTIAL OILS

Choose from:

Melissa oils (see page 60)

Cyprian oils (see page 82)

Nut Parchment oils (see page 82)

Pomander oils (see page 86)

Use 30 drops of any of the above oils for every 4oz of wax

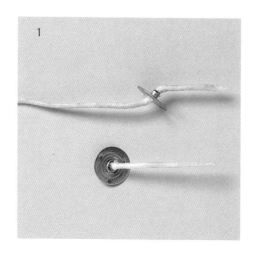

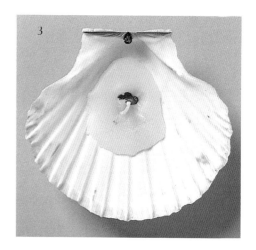

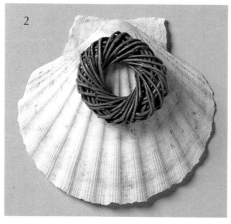

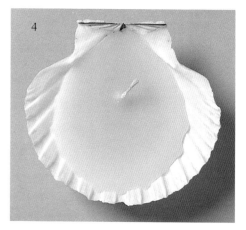

1. Wicks come in several sizes so choose one suited to the size of your shell. The depth of the candle does not affect the wick size. For extra-large shells use more than one wick. Dip a short length of wick into melted candle wax and leave it to dry and harden – do this only once. Thread the waxed wick through the hole in the base of the stabilizer until about 2in shows above the base; pull the wick through using a small pair of pliers. Clip off the bottom of the wick. Pinch shut the metal tube on the stabilizer at the base of the wick with the pliers.

2. Glue the base of the wicker ring to the curved underside of the scallop shell using strong, quick-drying glue or, preferably, a glue gun. Make sure that the shell sits level on the base and leave to set.

3. Melt old, broken candles or bought candle wax in an old metal saucepan. Melt the wax very slowly over a low flame or use a heat diffuser. If you are melting down old candles remove their wicks. When the melted wax has cooled a little and before it forms a skin add the oil mix and stir very gently. Stir the wax as little as possible to avoid air bubbles in the finished candle. Using a small, pre-warmed ladle, spoon a tablespoon of the warm, still-liquid scented wax carefully into the bottom of the shell. As the wax begins to skin over, place the stabilizer in the wax. Leave the wax to set cold.

4. Keep the wick vertical and use the ladle to fill up the shell with more scented liquid wax in stages. Do not fill the shell to the very top. Finished shell candles are shown opposite.

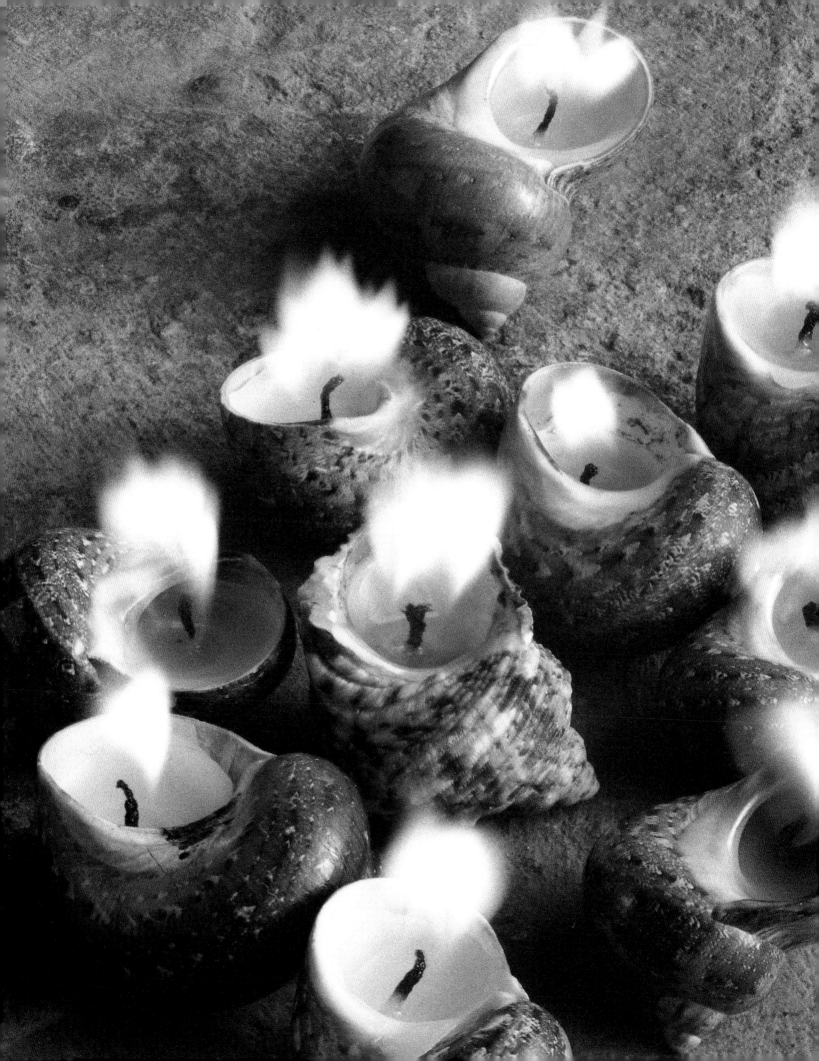

Pomander

Pomanders are a traditional aromatic delight. They are highly decorative hung from a ribbon or grouped together in bowls to form a fragrant centerpiece, and they are extremely simple to make. Seville or bitter oranges are the best choice as they are far more aromatic and less juicy than sweet oranges. Whole Seville oranges dry well for use in decorations, while other citrus fruits such as clementines and kumquats also make excellent smaller pomanders for use in wreaths and swags. Lemons and limes can also be used, but orange is more traditional. When you buy cloves for making a pomander you should select those with big heads for maximum visual impact. I have found that the best cloves can be found in oriental food shops where whole cloves are almost an everyday cooking ingredient. Pomanders are quite heavily scented, but if you wish to emphasize their fragrance still further you can paint the surface with oil of clove. Appropriately festive at Yuletide, try hanging pomanders on a Christmas tree or place them in a bowl close to a central-heating radiator where the steady warmth will draw out their spicy, citrus fragrance to best effect.

MATERIALS

Drafting or adhesive tape,
about $^1\!/_2$in wide
Seville orange
Cloves, whole
Ribbon, $^1\!/_2$in wide

EQUIPMENT

Wooden skewer, knitting needle or
wooden matchstick

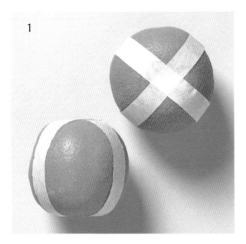

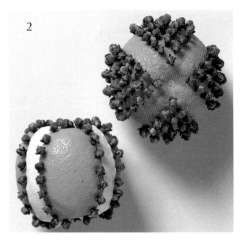

1. Cut two lengths of drafting or adhesive tape; each piece should be long enough to wrap once around the circumference of the orange with a small overlap. Stick the two lengths of tape to the skin of the Seville orange, dividing it into four equal segments.

2. Using a wooden skewer, a knitting needle or a wooden matchstick, prick even lines of holes in the skin of the orange, starting alongside the tape and keeping the holes approximately $^1\!/_4$in apart. Make the holes as deep as the stems of the cloves. Do not make too many holes at a time – no more than about six – as the skin of the orange closes up quite quickly and can then obscure the holes. Choose cloves with large heads. Push the whole cloves into the holes one by one, inserting them right up to their heads. As the orange dries it will shrink and the skin becomes taut, so bringing the holes slightly closer together which causes the cloves to stand up attractively just above the surface of the orange. Continue to make lines of holes and insert the cloves neatly until the entire exposed surface of the orange skin is covered. Remove the strips of tape.

Place the pomander in a warm, dry place such as inside an airing cupboard, on top of a central-heating boiler or on a radiator.

Turn the pomander over from time to time to make sure that it dries out evenly all around; this process should take three to four weeks. The cloves should act as a preservative and prevent the orange from going rotten.

When the orange has completely dried out, position two lengths of decorative ribbon over the gaps left by the tape. Tie the loose ends in a bow so that you can hang the pomander. For pomanders which are to be placed in bowls rather than hung, you can cover the whole orange with cloves, positioned either randomly or in neat lines.

There is an alternative method for making pomanders. When you have inserted all the cloves in the fruit you can cure the orange in a bowlful of mixed powders – for instance cinnamon, orris root, clove and allspice powders. Roll the orange in the mixed powders so that it is completely covered and leave it to dry out still in contact with the powders. The drying process can take up to six weeks. Although this is a tried and tested method for making pomanders, I find that using powders retards drying and is also rather messy. I would recommend that you follow the method described in steps 1 and 2 instead as the end result is more attractive. The finished pomanders are shown opposite.

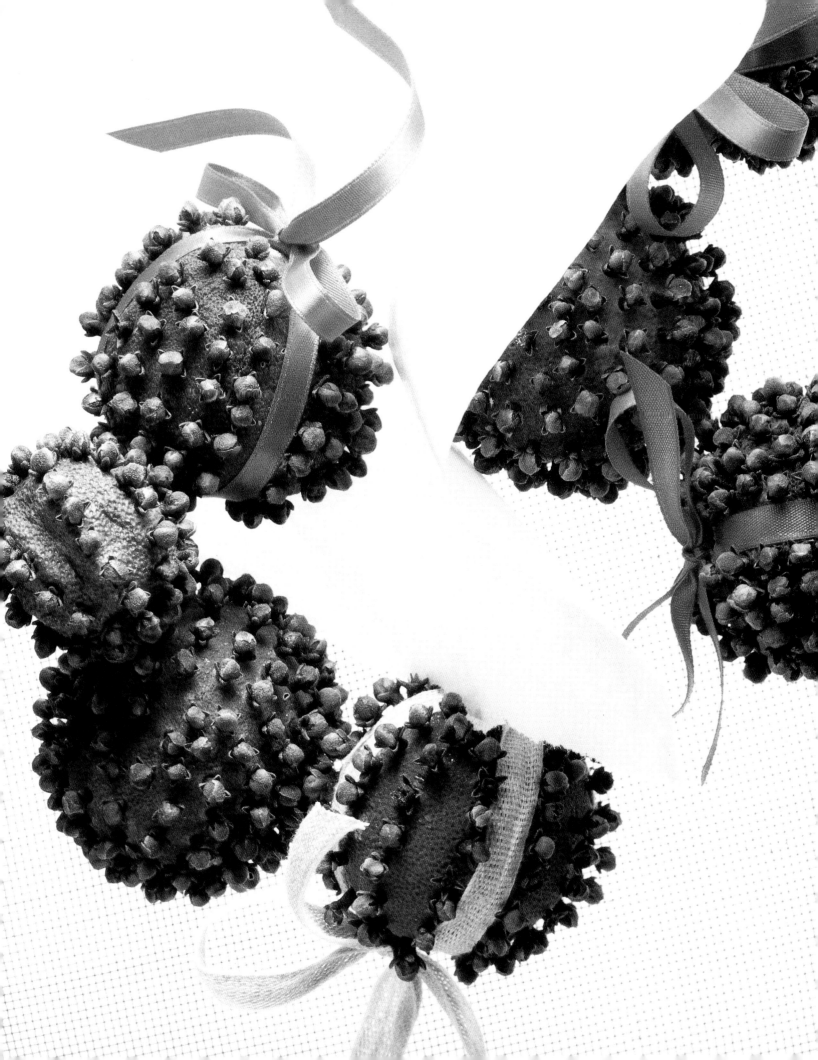

Writing Paper and Scented Inks

Letter-writing will take on a whole new dimension when you discover the delights of subtly scented writing papers and inks. To make your own fragrant, personalized notepapers, just right for those extra-special messages, follow the method described for scenting paper for lining drawers (see page 98.) As noted in the drawer liners project, paper takes up scent easily, but you should not apply oil directly to the paper as it will leave unsightly stains. For this reason it is best to perfume paper by "infection." This involves making a fabric sachet filled with a pot-pourri mixture. The paper and fabric sachet are then sealed together so that they are completely airtight and left for a few days for the scent to have time to impregnate the paper. If you wish to make scented inks, you should select suitably strong oils such as lavender, lemon grass or rosemary to have a noticeable effect. In addition, choose a brand of ink which has as little of its own scent as possible.

MATERIALS
Good-quality writing ink
Strongest proof vodka available

EQUIPMENT
Mixing bowls or bottles
Pipette
Small funnel
Decorative glass bottle with stopper

ESSENTIAL OILS
Since inks carry a certain amount of scent of their own, the effect of the oil will necessarily be slight, so use one distinctive perfume rather than a mix. See right for a list of suitable oils

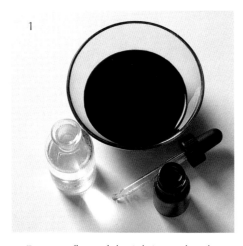

1. Decant 2fl oz of the ink into a bowl or a bottle. Prepare your chosen essential oil (see below) by accurately measuring out 100 drops into a glass vessel using a pipette.

In Britain the purchase of perfume alcohol requires a special licence and therefore it is not widely available. I suggest you use a high proof spirit such as vodka as a substitute. Measure out one teaspoonful of the strongest proof vodka that you can find and mix the essential oil and the vodka together in a glass vessel. It is vital that you mix the oil and the spirit together *before* you add the ink, otherwise the three will not blend. The vodka acts as a "solubolizer" which enables the ink and the essential oil to blend well together. Vodka is the most suitable spirit to use as it has no smell and so it will not interfere with the perfume provided by the essential oil. Add the essential oil and the spirit very slowly to the ink, a little at a time. If you

PURE ESSENTIAL OILS
Powerfully scented natural oils which will blend well with ink include:
Patchouli
Frankincense
Lemon grass
Cypress

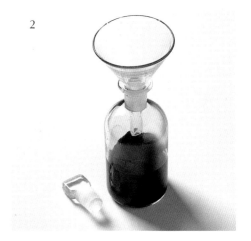

do not follow this order of blending, the mixture will separate and the results will look like a vinaigrette. If by any chance your scented ink mixture should separate, just shake up the bottle well before using it.

2. Decant the scented ink through a funnel into an attractive glass bottle with a stopper. Although it is quite possible to scent inks of any color, darker inks such as strong blue and black will give the most successful results. Because the addition of vodka and the drops of essential oil naturally dilute the ink, some paler inks may appear washed out and lose the impact of their original color when used. If you are combining perfumed inks with scented writing paper, then the two should preferably be scented with the same fragrance, otherwise the result may be an overpowering or unpleasant clash of scents. The finished scented inks and paper are shown in the photograph opposite.

SYNTHETIC OILS
The following synthetic blends are suitable oils for scenting inks:
Carnation-scented
Violet-scented
Magnolia-scented
Rose-scented

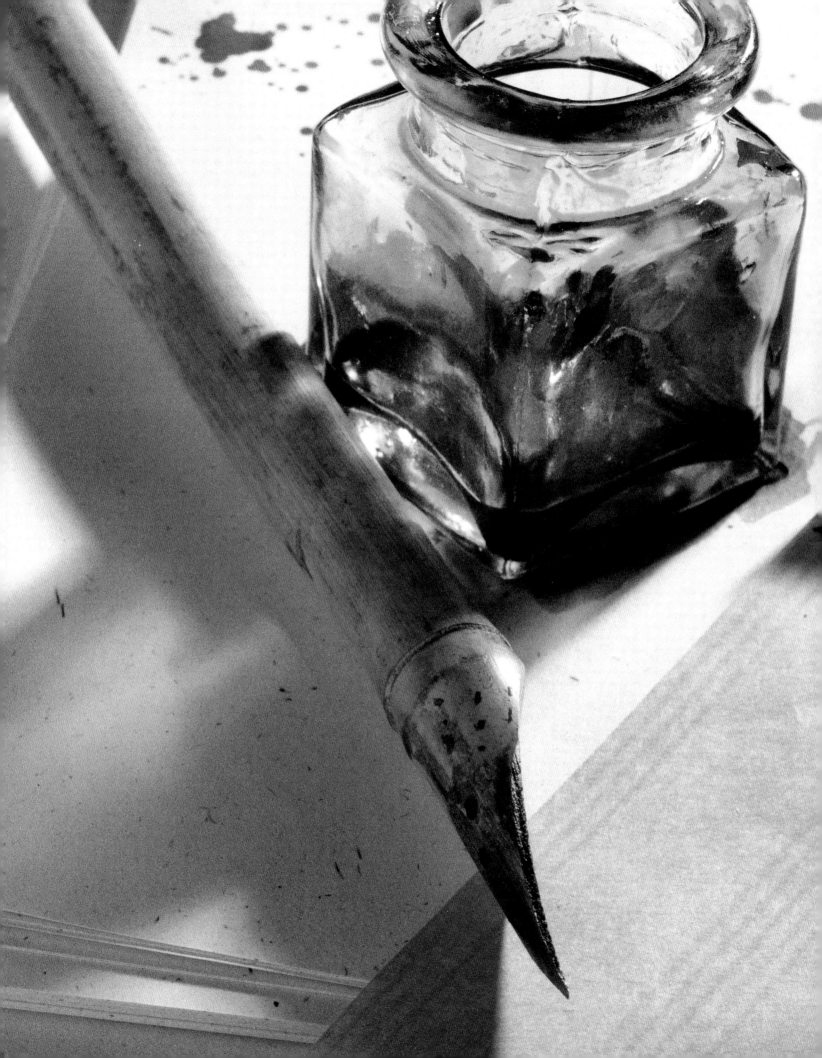

Furniture Polish

*T*o keep pieces of wooden furniture in good condition and at the same time till your home with fresh, herby scents such as rosemary, lavender or lemon grass, try preparing this rich beeswax furniture polish. It is quite simple to make and a pleasure to use. While bringing your furniture to a beautiful shine, it will exude its own particular perfume. As an added bonus, all the recommended oils are insect repellent. Stored in an airtight container in a dark place, the polish will keep fresh and fragrant for many months.

MATERIALS

8oz unrefined beeswax

2oz household soap

1 pint minimeral spirit (turpentine)

(Note that white spirit will not work)

1 pint water

EQUIPMENT

Coarse grater

Three mixing bowls

Bain-marie (double saucepan)

Heat-diffusing mat

Saucepan

Pipette

Airtight container (such as a

glass jar or cann with screw-top lid)

ESSENTIAL OILS

25 drops of any one of the following:

Cedarwood

Lavender

Lemon grass

Rosemary

Rosewood

If you wish to use any essential oils that are not on the above list, you should note that the scent must blend with the beeswax and mineral spirit

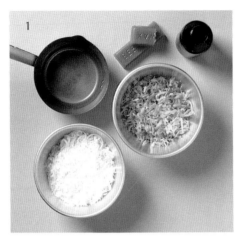

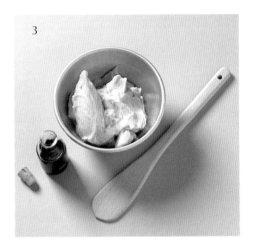

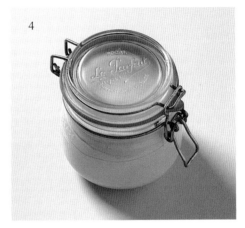

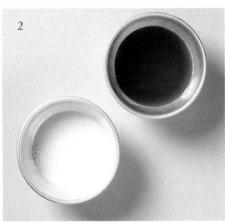

1. First assemble your materials. Grate the blocks of unrefined beeswax using an ordinary coarse cheese grater. Place the gratings in a bowl. Clean the grater and use it again to grate the soap; set aside the grated soap in another bowl. Measure out the required quantity of mineral spirit into a vessel and place 1 pint of water in a saucepan.

2. Dissolve the grated beeswax in the mineral spirit in the bain-marie (double saucepan) over a gentle heat, using the heat-diffusing mat. You should watch the melting mixture carefully all the time and do not allow the mineral spirit to get too hot and evaporate. Do not leave the pan unattended. Turn off the heat as soon as all the beeswax has melted. Next, dissolve the soap gratings in the water in a second saucepan.

3. When the beeswax mixture and the soap mixture are both melted to a liquid form (they will still be quite warm,) you can combine them together in a clean mixing bowl. Using a wooden spoon, blend the two liquids together in the bowl by stirring slowly and evenly. Continue to stir and blend together thoroughly until the mixture is almost cold. Use a pipette to add an accurate amount of your chosen essential oil and stir the oil thoroughly into the mixture.

4. As the mixture cools it thickens, forming a thick, creamy paste. Pour the mixture into an airtight container and leave it to harden overnight; do not yet seal. Only seal the container when the mixture has set. Store the polish in a dark place. The finished furniture polish is shown opposite.

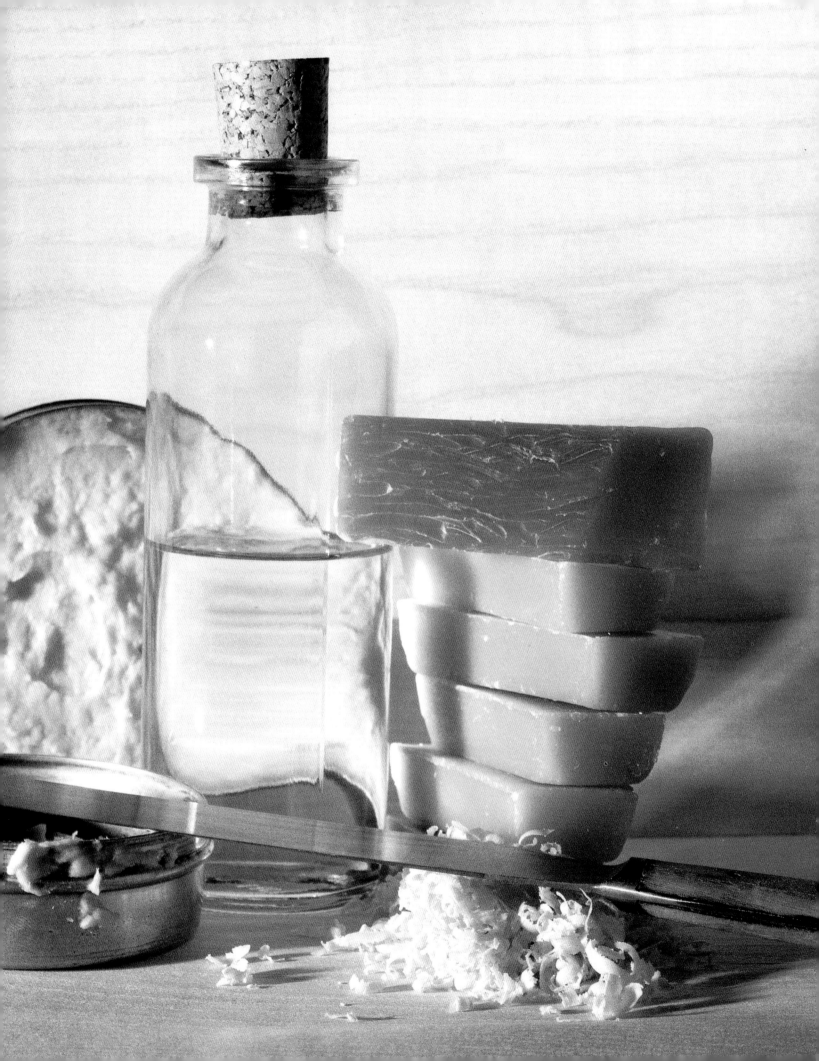

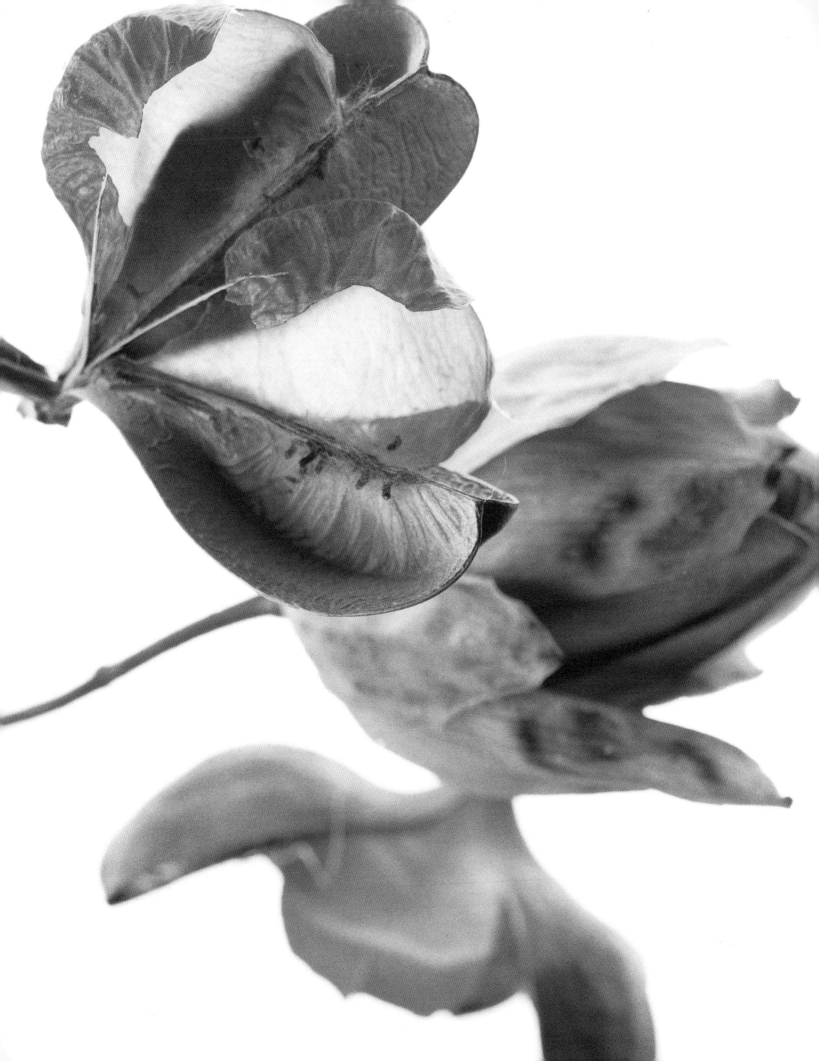

SCENTED DECORATIONS

DRIED FLOWERS ARE OFTEN THOUGHT OF AS AUTUMN OR FALL

AND WINTER DECORATION – SOMETHING OF A SUBSTITUTE FOR THE

SPRING AND SUMMER BLOOMS WE CAN ENJOY IN THEIR SEASON.

WITH THE WIDE RANGE OF FRESH AND DRIED PLANT MATERIAL

NOW AVAILABLE TO US THROUGHOUT THE YEAR, IT IS POSSIBLE TO

DRY ALL MANNER OF FLOWERS SUCCESSFULLY FOR USE IN FLORAL

DECORATIONS, SEE THE DRYING TECHNIQUES ON PAGES 24-29.

ONE ELEMENT OFTEN MISSING FROM DRIED FLOWER ARRANGE-

MENTS IS SCENT, BUT THE FOLLOWING PROJECTS INCLUDE ADVICE

FOR PERFUMING WITH ESSENTIAL OILS AND PERFUME BLENDS.

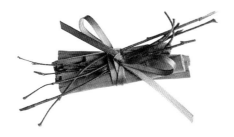

Mossy Spring Wreath

*T*his mossy springtime wreath is scented with the oils used in the Primavera mix, see page 60. Constructed on a wire wreath base, it evokes the sights and smells of the early year, as the first flowers appear through their winter covering of mosses, ivy and leaves. The flowers, in spring shades of yellow and blue, are all dried in silica, see page 28. Choose double-flowered varieties of daffodils, parrot tulips, lilies and polyanthus and dry the flower heads only, leaving just a short stem to be wired or glued to the ring. You can hang the wreath on a door, a wall or above a fireplace, or lay it horizontally as a table decoration.

MATERIALS

16in diameter wire wreath

Sack or sphagnum moss

Carpet moss

Florist's reel wire

One 12in of 18swg florist's wire for the loop

Pussy willow twigs

Ivy sprigs, glycerined

Silica-dried flowers: double daffodils, parrot tulips, yellow lilies, yellow and blue polyanthus, purple hellebores, miniature daffodils (eg 'Sol d'Or')

7in lengths of 22swg florist's ready-cut (stub) wire for wiring

Eucalyptus leaves, dried or glycerined

EQUIPMENT

Glue gun

Mossing pins

Poultry roasting bag

ESSENTIAL OIL MIX

Primavera mix

(see page 60)

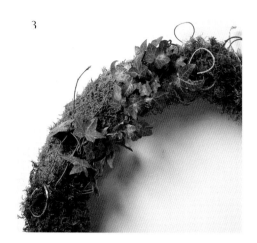

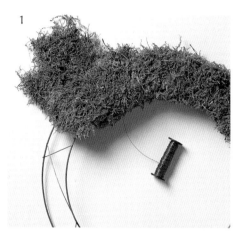

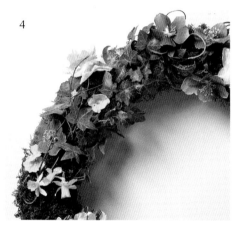

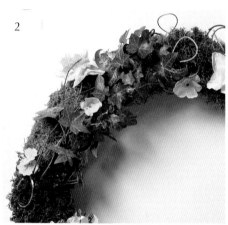

1. Start to fill the wreath base with moss. Use clumps of sack or sphagnum moss to fill the inside of the base; secure it by winding reel wire around the moss as you go. Cover the outside of the base with sheets of carpet moss; secure it in the same way.

2. Complete the mossing and aim to keep the covering even all around the ring. To make a loop to hang the ring, bend the 18swg florist's wire in half and pass it through the back of the wire base. Twist it to make a firm, circular loop and tuck the ends of the wire into the moss. Begin to add plant material to the ring, starting with the pussy willow twigs. Secure them to the ring by pushing them under the florist's reel wire used to bind the moss. Add small clumps of carpet moss to support the smaller flowers.

Secure with the glue gun and mossing pins. Add several sprigs of the glycerined ivy to give movement to the arrangement; secure with the glue gun and mossing pins.

3. Begin to infill with the daffodils, tulips and polyanthus. Those which have been wired (for wiring see pages 128-9) are secured by their wires; other flowers are attached to the ring using the glue gun.

4. Add the hellebore flowers, grouping them together. Then add the lilies, more polyanthus and the miniature daffodils. Finally, add sprigs of eucalyptus. Distribute 30 drops of the essential oil mix around the moss and seal the whole arrangement in a poultry roasting bag (or acrylic sheeting) for 24 hours to take up the scent. The finished mossy spring wreath is shown opposite.

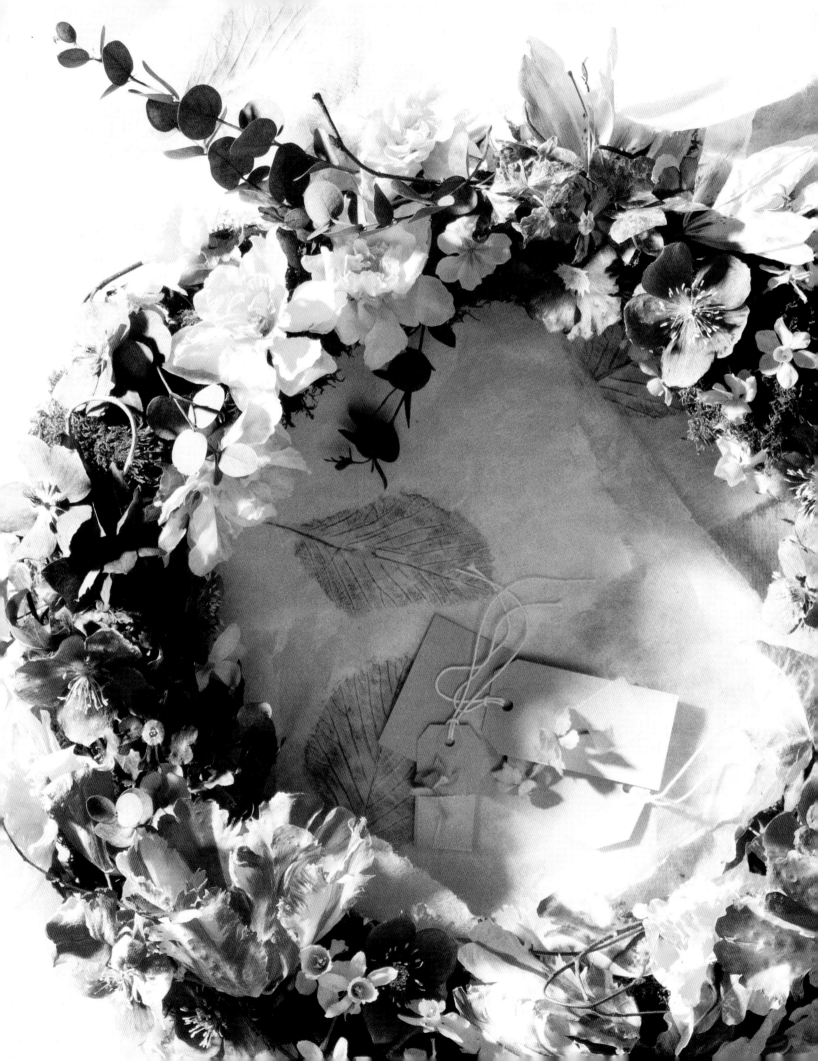

Scented Summer Circle

To conjure up the spirit of mid-summer huge, blowsy double pink peonies are the main focus of my scented circle. The luscious flowers nestle in a bed of oakmoss and eucalyptus leaves and are surrounded by old-fashioned roses in deep pink, hybrid tea roses and dark red rosebuds dotted here and there. The pinks and gray-greens contrast with a few sprigs of purple-blue larkspur. The circle is richly scented to evoke the fragrance of a garden in high summer.

MATERIALS

Oakmoss (or other moss)
14in diameter dry foam ring
Massing pins, hairpins or hooped 7in lengths of 22swg florist's ready-cut (stub) wire
14in length of 18swg florist's ready-cut (stub) wire
Eucalyptus leaves, glycerined
Five large, pale pink double peonies, dried in silica
Air-dried flowers: green-blue hydrangeas, old-fashioned pink roses, miniature red rosebuds and sprigs of purple-blue larkspur
Pale pink hybrid tea roses, silica dried
Ribbon to hang

EQUIPMENT

Shallow dish
Kitchen paper
Sharp knife
Glue gun
Poultry roasting bag

ESSENTIAL OIL MIX

Chinese Peony mix (see page 70) or
Shalimar mix (see page 70) or
Old English Rose mix (see page 72)

1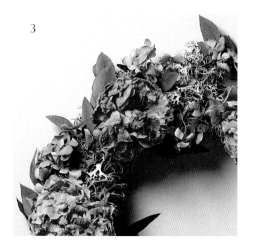

2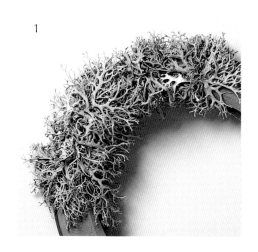

3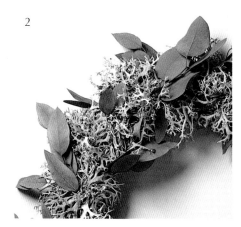

4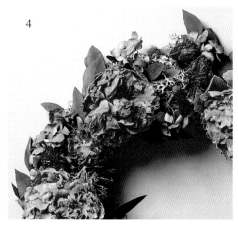

1. Soak the oakmoss in a shallow dish of water to freshen the color and make the moss pliable for working. Squeeze the water from the moss and pat semi-dry with kitchen paper. Round off the square edges of the foam ring with a sharp knife.

To make a loop to hang the ring, push the end of the 18swg florist's wire through the foam above the plastic so that about 2in sticks out into the middle of the ring. Bend down the long end of the wire under the plastic base and twist it around the short end to secure; tuck the ends into the foam. Twist the loop of wire around itself to form a smaller, circular loop for attaching the ribbon to hang up the finished ring. Begin to cover the ring with the oakmoss, securing it with mossing pins and the glue gun.

2. Complete the mossing. Position the dried eucalyptus leaves so they face in different directions; secure them with the glue gun.

3. Place the five peony flowers on the ring, spacing them evenly. Place dried heads of hydrangea flowers and old-fashioned pink roses in between the peonies; secure the flowers with the glue gun.

4. Fill in the gaps with more flowers, clustering the hybrid tea roses and the rosebuds in groups and securing with the glue gun. Finally, attach a few sprigs of larkspur for a cool contrast and add a few more eucalyptus leaves. Distribute 30 drops of the essential oil mix around the moss and seal the whole arrangement in a poultry roasting bag for 24 hours to take up the scent. The finished scented summer circle is shown opposite.

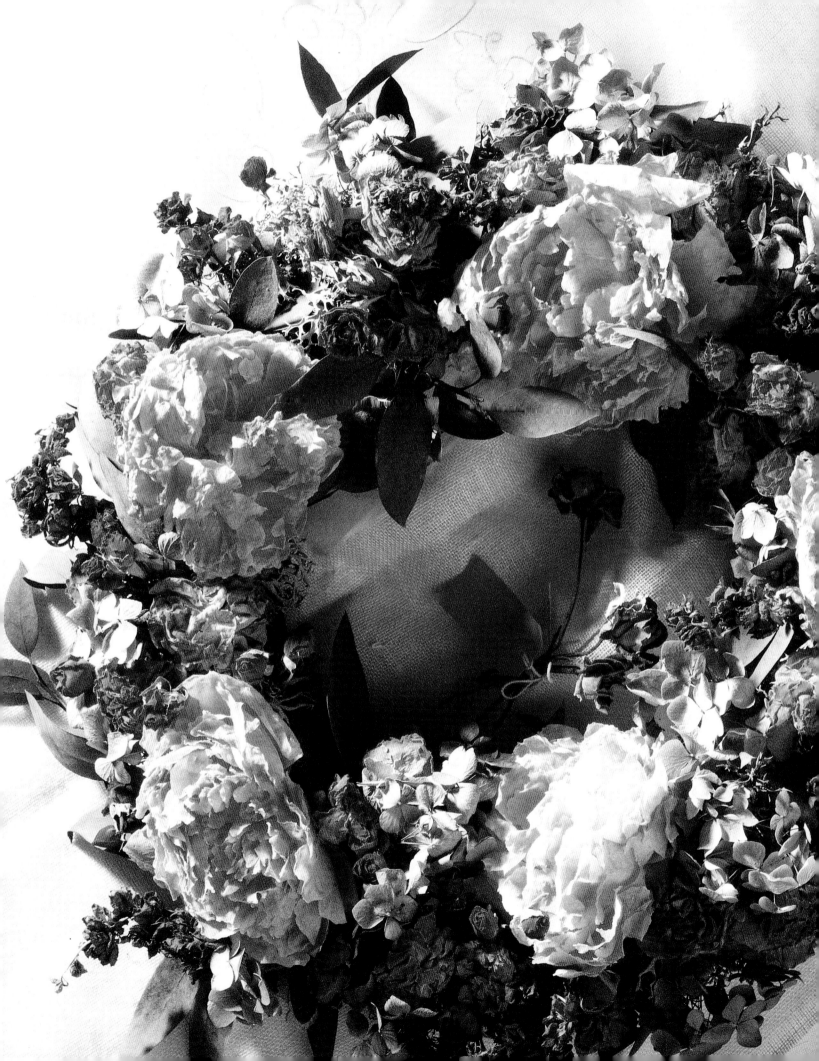

Spicy Mulling Ring

*T*his mulling ring carries the spicy scents of cinnamon, clove, allspice and orange and evokes the rich, woody aromas and deepening colors of the onset of fall. The small muslin bags of spices and bundles of cinnamon sticks detach from the ring for use in mulled drinks. Coils of orange peel add highlights to the arrangement. These are easy to dry (leave plenty of pith on them to prevent them snapping) placed on a radiator or in an airing cupboard. To give the ring added spice, rub the whole nutmegs with a Q-tip dipped in essential oils to shine and darken the surface and yield a delicious fragrance.

MATERIALS

12in unpeeled willow ring

10in length of 18swg wire

Long pieces of sweet orange peel, dried

Nutmegs, whole

Star anise

Ginger roots, dried whole

Mace, whole

8 x 20in cream muslin

1 tablespoon each of crushed cloves and cinnamon and ground nutmeg

10 cloves, whole

18 cinnamon sticks, whole

7in lengths of 22swg florist's ready-cut (stub) wire

Ribbon

EQUIPMENT

Glue gun

cotton bud or scrap of cloth

ESSENTIAL OIL MIX

10 drops orange

10 drops cinnamon

5 drops clove

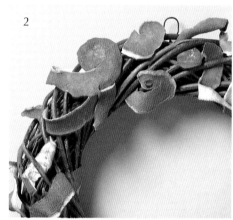

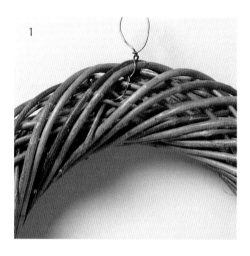

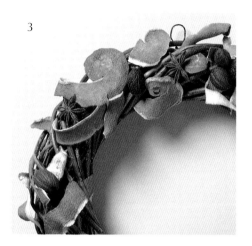

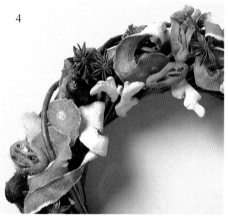

1. Bend the length of 18swg florist's wire in half and thread it through the willow ring, twisting it into a loop to hang the ring. Tuck the ends of the wire well into the body of the ring. Make sure you complete this step now as it is difficult to add the wire loop later.

2. Thread pieces of dried orange peel through the ring; distribute them evenly.

3. Add the whole nutmegs in pairs or threes, securing them with the glue gun. Begin to add the star anise and other plant material, distributing it evenly to form a pleasing arrangement. Group the small items together for extra visual impact.

4. Continue to build up the plant material around the ring until you are satisfied with the density of the arrangement. Add whole dried ginger roots, mace, nutmegs, star anise

and a few more pieces of orange peel. Secure all the items to the ring with the glue gun. Finally, add little muslin spice bags and bundles of cinnamon sticks to the ring. For the spice bag, cut out a circle of muslin 4in in diameter and place a small heap of crushed spices in the middle. Gather up the muslin, bunch into a bag and tie with thread or ribbon. Stick a whole clove into the bottom for decoration. Secure to the ring with a length of 22swg florist's wire. For the cinnamon bundles, break whole sticks into 3in lengths and tie three pieces into a bundle with ribbon. Make six bundles and secure to the ring with the glue gun. With a Q-tip, rub the essential oil over the nutmegs, orange peel and star anise. The finished mulling ring is shown opposite.

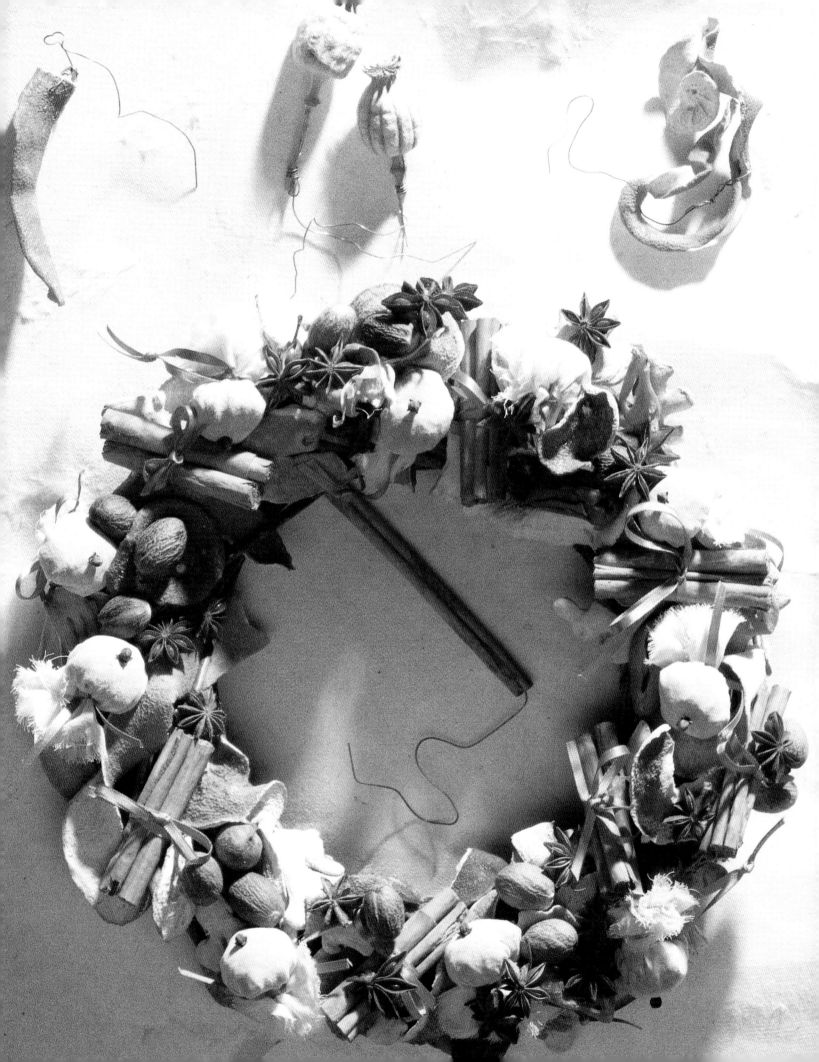

Chistmas Candelabra

I used an interesting range of plant material to create this festive Christmas hanging candelabra. The apple rings, which are so much a feature of the arrangement, are quite easy to dry. Choose large apples with red skins, slice them and spread them out to dry on a radiator or a central-heating boiler. They will be ready in about two days. Make sure that you never leave the candles on the wreath unattended when lit. Replace the candles when they burn down to within 2in of their holders. Use a Q-tip to polish the leaf surfaces with aromatic oils to add a warm, rich and spicy scent to the arrangement.

MATERIALS

Three plastic candle holders
Gold spray paint
14in diameter vine
or twig wreath
22swg) florist's wire
10ft of cinnamon-colored
ribbon½in wide
Three candles to fit the holders
Portugal laurel leaves, glycerined
Clematis seedheads, glycerined
Locust beans, dried
Tree peony seedheads, dried
Apple slices, dried
Miniature pomegranates, dried
Poppy seedheads, dried
Half walnuts, sprayed gold

EQUIPMENT

Glue gun
Q-tip

ESSENTIAL OIL MIXES

Festival oil mix (see page 54) or
Zanzibar oil mix (see page 86)

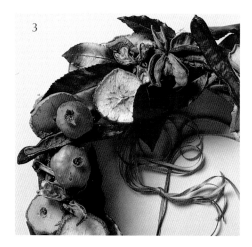

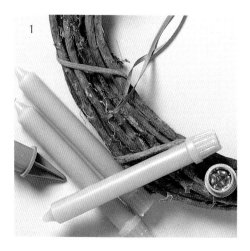

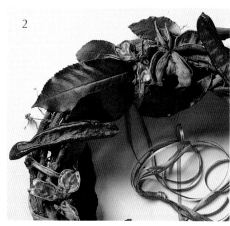

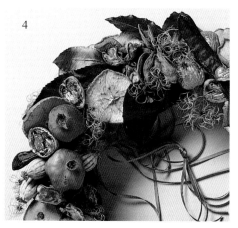

1. Spray the candle holders and the walnut halves gold and leave to dry. Find three well-spaced points on the wreath to insert the candle holders. Wedge them into the wreath; secure with glue and 22swg florist's wire when quite vertical. Cut three lengths of ribbon, each about 40in long. Double the lengths over and thread the looped ends through the wreath at three points, midway between a pair of candle holders. Thread the cut ends of each length through the looped end and pull through to secure the ribbon to the wreath. Tie all six cut ends together and check by holding up the cut ends that the wreath hangs horizontally from the knot.

2. With the candle holders attached, turn the wreath upside down to rest on the candle holders. Make an "outline" of laurel leaves.

Then glue the leaves into place. Glue five dried tree peony seedheads and a few dried locust beans to the wreath; they should be distributed evenly among the laurel leaves.

3. Continue to add dried plant material. Arrange it evenly around the wreath and secure using the glue gun. Add the dried apple slices and miniature pomegranates in the same way, gluing them into position.

4. Add the poppy seedheads – singly and in pairs – and the half walnuts; wire them into position and fill any gaps in the arrangement. Add some sprays of clematis seedheads. Use a Q-tip to polish the leaves with the essential oil mix. Turn the wreath the right way up, insert the candles and hang the ring from the ribbons. The finished Christmas Candelabra is shown opposite.

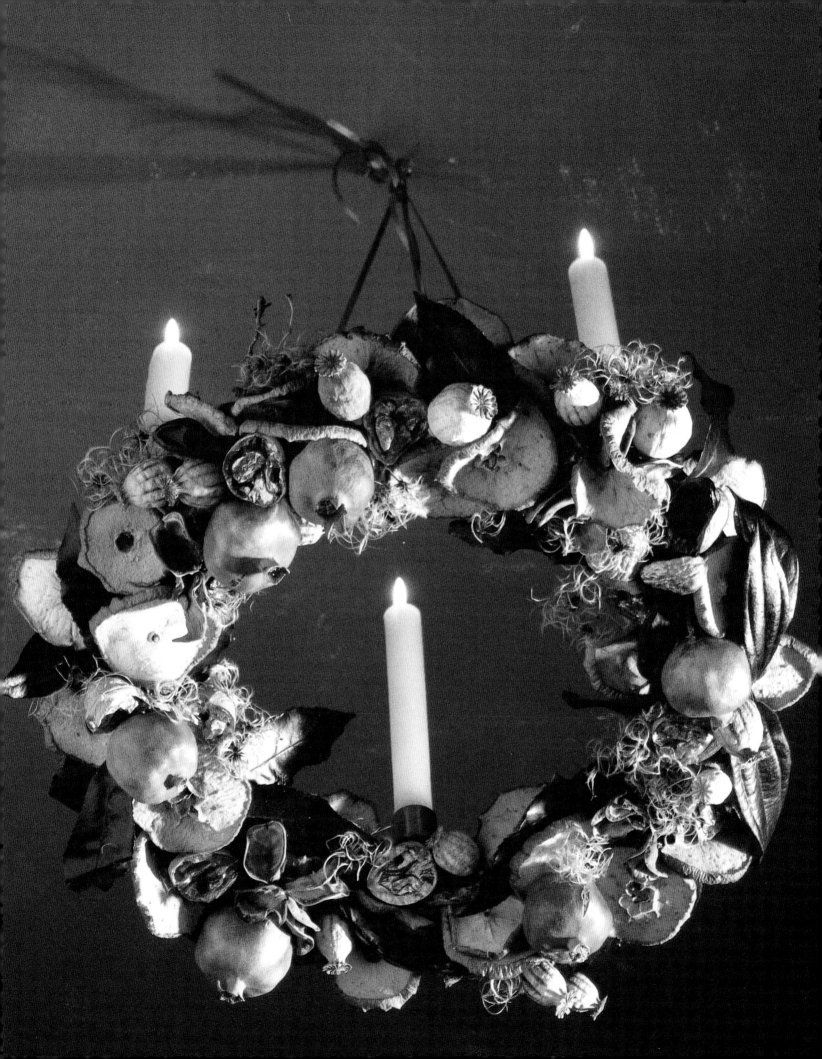

Shell Drop

*T*he beautiful sculptural quality of shells make them a delight to work with. Here I tried to give an impression of shells left piled up on the seashore by the tide by positioning the various types of shells in different directions. To create this unusual swag, gather shells, driftwood, seaweeds, flotsam and jetsam on your next visit to the seaside and impregnate them with the woody, spicy scent of the Cyprian mix given on page 82. Combine marine material with parched plant material such as pine cones sprayed white, seedheads and lichens.

MATERIALS

4ft x 3½in x ½in wooden baseboard

Two brass mirror plates and screws

Two screws and rawl plugs, to hang the finished piece on the wall

14in length of 18swg wire

7in lengths of florist's ready-cut (stub) wire for the loops

Florist's tape

Piece of 4ft 6in x 14in florist's 2in wire netting or garden wire mesh

Carpet or sphagnum moss

Florist's reel wire

Shells, all kinds of types and sizes

Oakmoss

Miniature lotus seedheads

EQUIPMENT

Screwdriver

Stapler or staple gun

Scissors

Electric drill

Acrylic sheeting

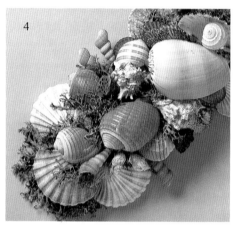

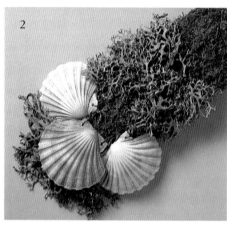

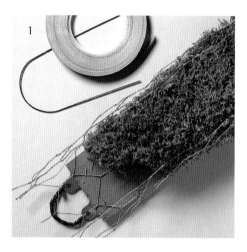

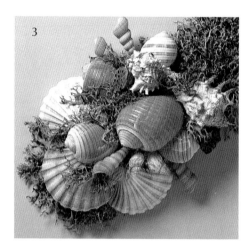

1. Screw the brass mirror plates to the back of the wooden baseboard at one short end to hang the arrangement. Thread the length of 18swg wire through the holes in the mirror plates; twist firmly to form a thick loop and cover with florist's tape. Lay the wire netting centrally over the front of the baseboard, with an equal overlap at each end. Secure the netting firmly to the board with staples. Lay the moss thickly down the middle of the baseboard and tuck over the two long sides of the netting. The moss covering should be about 6in wide and 2in thick.

2. Turn the 3in of netting at each short end of the mossed base over and push the sharp ends into the moss. Turn the long sides of the netting into the middle, overlapping them by approximately 2in.

"Stitch" the netting with reel wire to form the base for the shells. Drill a small hole in the heavy shells for wiring. Start with three scallop shells and work from the bottom of the swag upward, interspersing the oakmoss.

3. Having decided on a mixed shell design about 10in long, start to wire and glue the shells to the mossed base. Continue to arrange and secure the shells in sections.

4. Arrange larger shells under the smaller ones. The smaller shells are simply glued on top. Complete the decoration with a crest of flat scallop shells at the top. Infill gaps with lotus seedheads, oakmoss or small shells. Distribute 100 drops of the essential oil mix on the oakmoss. Put the whole in acrylic sheeting for a few days to absorb the scent. The finished shell drop is shown opposite.

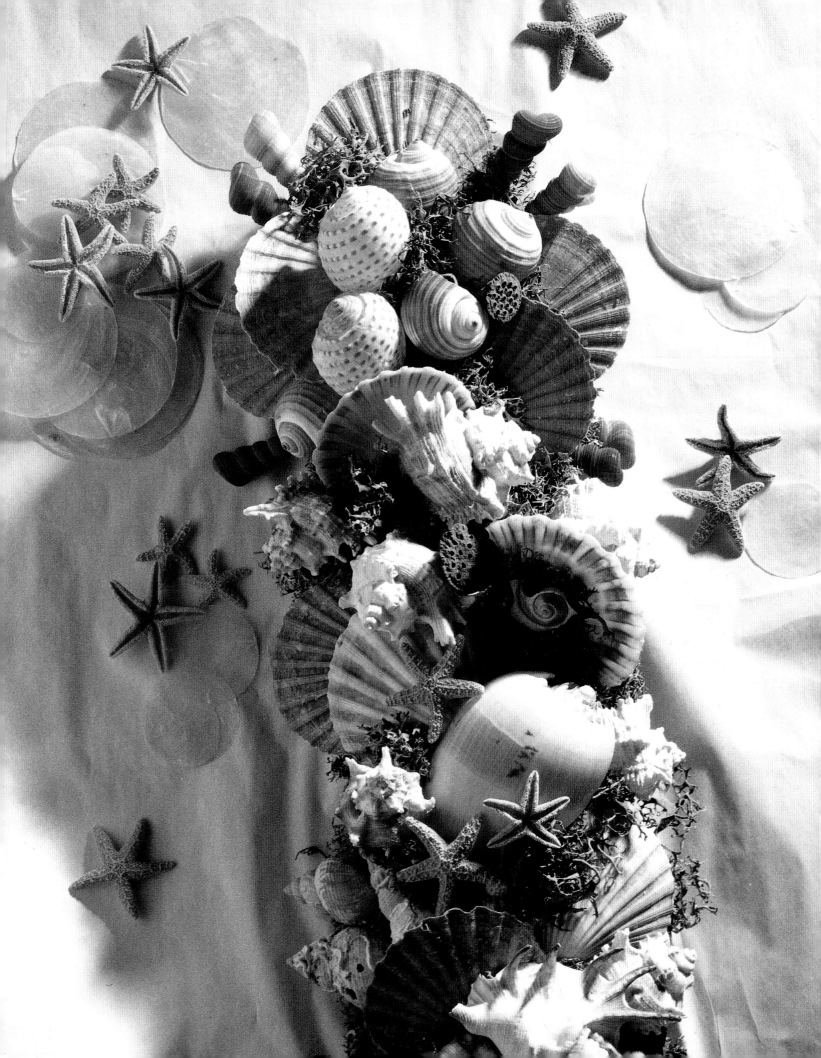

Hydrangea Garland

A garland with a fresh, floral scent provides spectacular decoration for all kinds of special occasions. Although this project requires quite a large amount of plant material, it is not too difficult to make. Flexible and versatile, this enchanting garland in fact consists of a continuous chain of dried flowers. You can make it to any length, working in short sections if you prefer, and then joining the sections together using wire covered with ribbon or cord. You could display this lavish chain of dried flowers over a doorway or a mirror, hung above a fireplace, draped along a beam or perhaps have it snaking down the middle of a dining table or looped along the front of a buffet for a party.

MATERIALS

10in lengths of 22swg florist's ready-cut (stub) wire

Hydrangeas, air dried

Mugwort, air dried

Small pink roses, air dried

Anaphalis, air dried

Eucalyptus leaves, glycerined

Myrtle leaves, glycerined

Soft cotton cord or good-quality silk ribbon with a wired edge

Florist's reel wire

EQUIPMENT

Florist's scissors or wire cutters

Sharp scissors for the cord or ribbon

Acrylic sheeting

ESSENTIAL OILS

Lavender or

Geranium or

Rose or

Bergamot

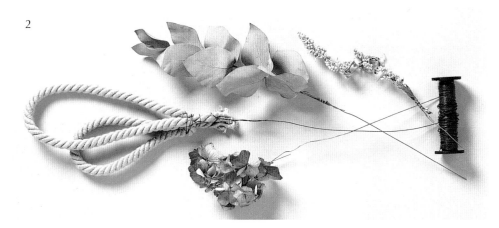

1

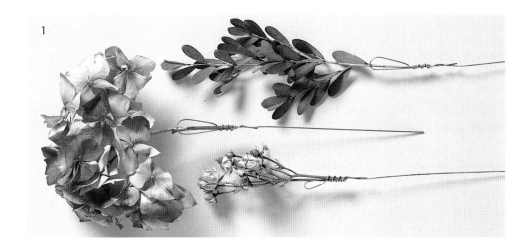

2

1. The secret to making this garland lies in mastering the technique of wiring. All the flowers and foliage are wired in the same way. First, you should practice wiring if you have not done it before. To wire the plant material, start by taking a small sprig of, for example, hydrangea and cut off the stem to approximately 2in. Bend the top 1½in of a piece of 7-in long piece of 22swg florist's stub wire into a U-shape. Lay the U end of the wire against the cut stem. The short end of the U-shaped wire should be roughly ½in longer than the cut stem. Bend the short end of the wire around the stem and bend the long end of the wire around the stem *and* the short end of wire several times to secure all together. The long end of wire now constitutes the stem.

Straighten this and wind it around the central core of reel wire to attach the sprig or spray to the garland. All the plant material is attached to the garland in this way.

2. Before starting work on the garland, decide how long you want it to be and cut a length of florist's reel wire to this length, allowing an extra 6in for binding on the end sprigs and the loops of cord or ribbon. Cut two lengths of soft cotton cord or ribbon, one 15in and the other 12in long. Fold each one into a loop. Bunch the four cut ends together and bind them tightly with one end of the length of reel wire. Follow the wiring technique explained to do this. In other words, bend the first 1½in of the reel wire into a U-shape and lay it along the cut ends of the cord or ribbon. Then bend the long end

3

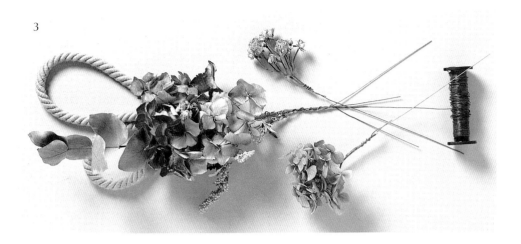

4

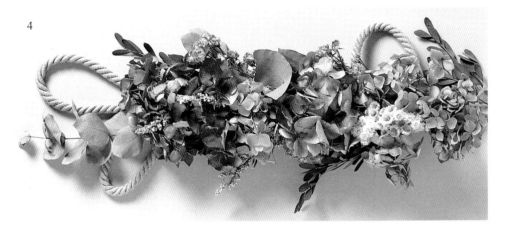

4. Continue to build up the garland in the same way, by twisting wired sprigs of flowers or foliage on to the central length of reel wire, adding sprigs of myrtle, a bunch of roses, more hydrangeas and contrasting sprigs of anaphalis. When you reach a point about 8in along the garland, wire on a single loop of cotton cord or ribbon to vary the texture of the growing garland.

Continue to lengthen the garland, varying the tones of the plant material so that the composition of the arrangement does not look too repetitive. Add more single loops of cord or ribbon at approximately 8in intervals on alternate sides of the garland for decoration and textural contrast. I suggest you do not cut the reel wire until you have added all the plant material you require to the garland and it has achieved its required overall length. However, if you find it easier to work the garland in short sections you can wire the sections together at the end.

When the garland has reached the required length, finish off the tail end by matching the plant material wired to the starting end. Make a similar grouping of hydrangea, eucalyptus and mugwort to that used at the beginning, but wired on in the *opposite* direction to the rest of the garland on a final double loop of cord or ribbon. Only at this point do you alter the direction of the plant material, to provide a neat finish.

To perfume a garland that is roughly 5ft long distribute 100 drops of the essential oil evenly around the garland (use proportionately more oil if the garland is longer than this,) then wrap the whole arrangement in acrylic sheeting for a day or two to take up the scent. The finished hydrangea garland is shown overleaf.

around all the cut cord ends and the short end of reel wire to secure well. The length of reel wire will form the core or flexible backbone of the garland. Do *not* cut the length of reel wire – it must run the length of the garland as all the sprays of flowers and leaves will be attached to it.

The success of this garland depends on its flexibility. Because dried plant material is often brittle, it is liable to break when handled or arranged. The wiring replaces fragile stems with something more pliable; it gives the dried plant material greater strength and simply by bending the wire in the required direction you can position the sprays exactly as you wish. Without wiring, the garland would lack movement and grace and much of the plant material would be damaged.

3. Lay a wired eucalyptus sprig in the middle of the two end loops of cotton cord or ribbon and add several wired sprigs of hydrangea, a few of mugwort and one of small pink roses. Twist the ends of all the wires together around the central length of florist's reel wire: the core of the garland. It is helpful to prepare several wired sprays of plant material in advance. Position the next few wired sprigs alongside the already attached sprigs to help you visualize how the garland will develop. When you are happy with the combination of colors and the juxtaposition of shape and density of flowers and leaf, attach the wired sprigs to the central length of reel wire. It is essential to keep all the flowers and foliage facing in the same direction, otherwise the finished garland will look messy.

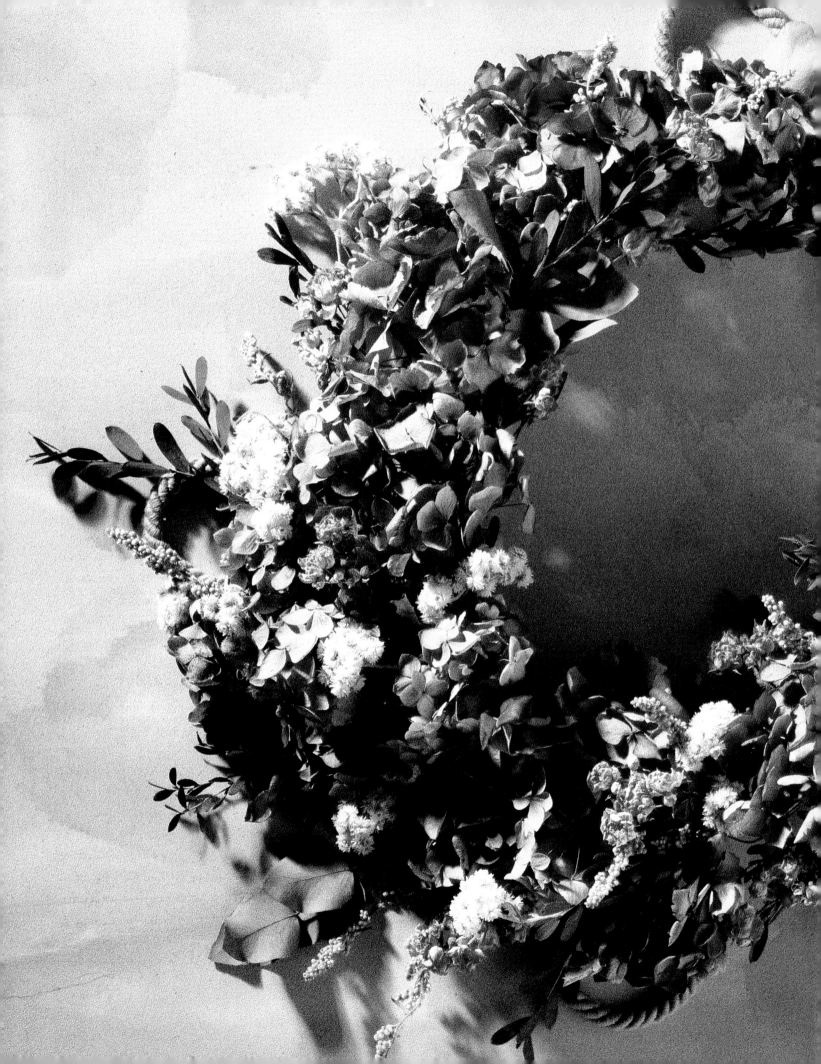

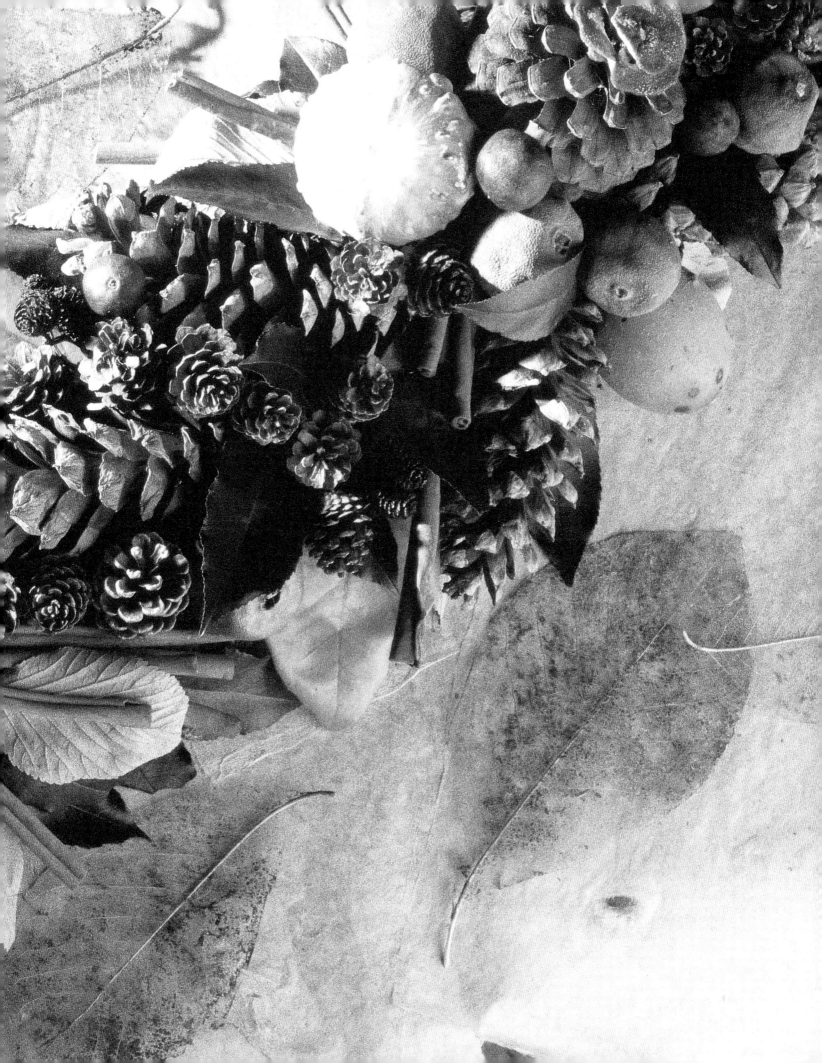

TOOLS & CONSTRUCTION

The pieces of floristry equipment that are illustrated opposite are useful tools for making the projects featured on pages 92-131. By acquiring some of these items I hope that you will find the process of constructing your own scented decorations both easy and enjoyable.

1. FOAM RING

Styrofoam rings are available in various sizes and are contained in a rigid plastic base. They are invaluable for making both fresh and dry flower arrangements. When working with dry plant material use a dry foam base; with fresh flowers the foam must be soaked until it has absorbed water. Foam bases are available in balls, cones and other forms.

2. WIRE-EDGED RIBBON

There are all sorts of wire-edged ribbons now on the market, ranging from the fairly narrow gauzy ribbon illustrated here, which is 1½in wide, to much heavier brocade and lamé ribbons of 3-4in width which are very useful for embellishing rings and swags. The wire edges allow you to shape and sculpt the ribbon beautifully.

3. FLORIST'S WIRES

Florist's or stub wires are the key to successful dry and fresh flower arranging. Dried flowers have rigid stems that lack movement. Wiring the stems gives more flexibility when creating an arrangement and enables you to position flowers as you want them. Wires come in different grades or thicknesses, from heavy wires for wiring weighty items such as cones, fruits and vegetables to the finest threadlike rose wires suitable for wiring light and delicate flowers and florets. (Note that "swg" stands for standard wire gauge.)

4. CANDLE HOLDERS

Sturdy plastic flameproof candle holders are invaluable when you come to making table decorations that combine candles with fresh or dried flowers. The spike on the holder grips firmly in the foam base and the whole keeps the candles upright and steady. Position the candle holders before you start to arrange the flowers; the base can then be disguised with leaves or flowers. Always blow out the candles before they burn down to the plant material. You should never leave candles burning unattended.

5. TWINE

It is well worth building up a collection of interesting twines and string which will be endlessly useful for all sorts of floral work such as tying bunches, making hanging loops and tying on labels.

6. FLORIST'S SCISSORS

A pair of sharp, well-made scissors is vital for all flower work; the scissors should be able to cut through tough stems and florist's wire.

7. SECATEURS

In order to cut through tough stems and branches or heavy-grade florist's wire a pair of secateurs is useful. Secateurs are also valuable in the garden for gathering leaves and branches for glycerining.

8. MOSSING PINS

Also known as German pins, these little loops of wire are obtainable from florist's retail outlets. However, if you cannot buy them ready-made you can easily make them yourself from short lengths of heavy-grade florist's wire bent into a loop; or just use a bobbypin instead! Use the pins to secure moss to a base or to pin stems and flowers in position on a swag or wreath base.

9. GLUE GUN

The invention of the glue gun has transformed much of modern floristry. The gun is invaluable for mossing a base and speeds up all forms of decorative flower work, whether you are using dried or fresh plant material. It is particularly useful when creating dried flower swags, rings and garlands. The gun works by heating and melting special glue sticks. You must allow the gun to cool completely after use before storing it away.

10. GUTTA TAPE

Thin, pliable gutta tape is much used by florists for winding around unsightly pieces of wire, particularly if the stub wire completely replaces the stem of the flower. Gutta tape is also useful for covering and softening hanging wires on rings, swags and garlands to prevent scratching.

11. REEL WIRE

This type of florist's wire comes in several grades or thicknesses; the most useful is the medium-grade wire. Reel wire is a continuous, flexible length of wire wound on to a bobbin. It is useful for making garlands and also for "stitching" wire netting.

12. WIRE CUTTERS

Although you can cut wires with strong scissors, this tends to blunt them quickly. A pair of wire cutters is a useful addition to your tool box, especially if you are using heavy-grade wires for large-scale arrangements.

13. RIBBONS

All types and widths of ribbon can be used in a hundred different ways to support and enhance flower decorations. It is useful to collect pieces of ribbon. I often make use of the very narrow ¼in cinnamon satin ribbon that is shown here.

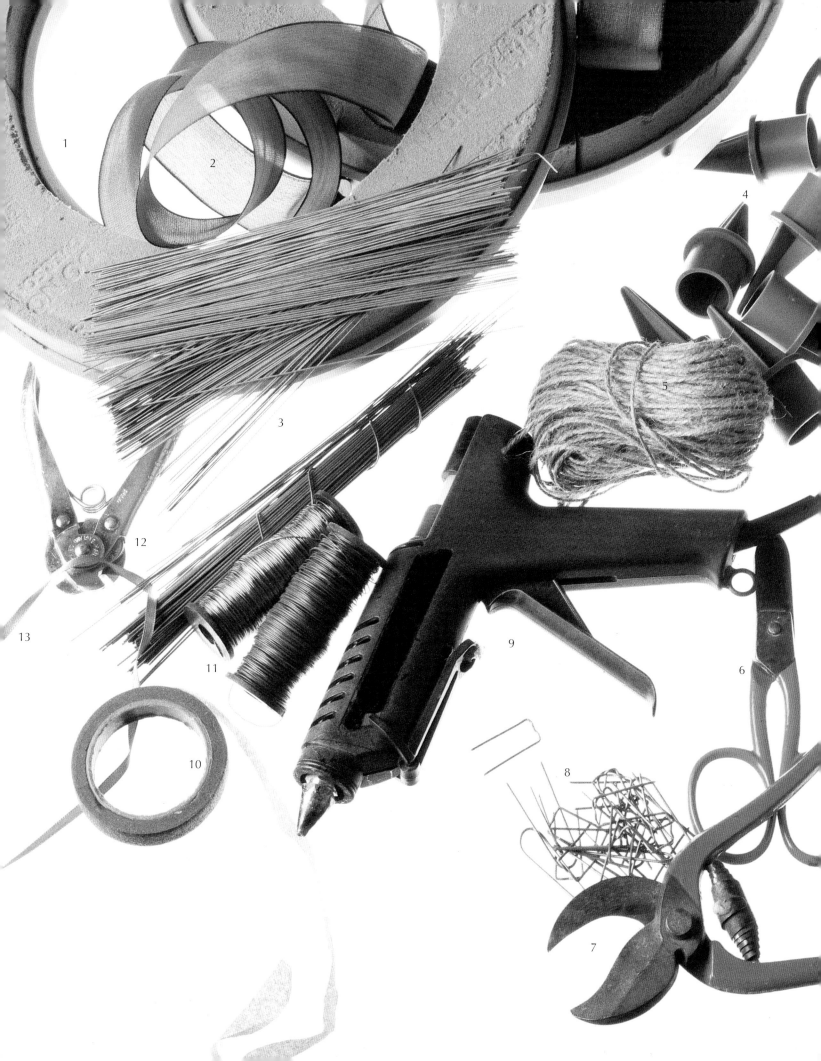

PLANT GAZETTEER

The plant gazetteer provides a quick botanical reference to the many plants in the book. It is listed in order of Latin names. Each entry gives the common name, followed by a brief description of the most useful parts of the plant (whether flowers, foliage, buds, roots etc) and suggestions for its use in the context of scented dried flower arranging.

Acacia dealbata
Mimosa
Fluffy, brilliant yellow flowers that grow up a slender stem. The leaves are fern-like and gray-green. Hang upside-down to air dry, or water dry. Lovely in spring pot-pourris.

Acer pseudoplatanus
Sycamore
Tree with bright-green leaves with five lobes that turn yellow in fall. The "windmill" seeds air dry flat and are decorative in pot-pourris.

Achillea filipendulina
Yarrow
Flat heads of compact clusters of small yellow flowers. To dry the florets should be fully open and the head firm. Hang upside-down to air dry in bunches. Keep color well. Use in lemony spring and summer pot-pourris.

Agastache mexicana
Agastache
Fragrant white or blue flowers in spikes. Hang upside-down to air dry. Use the leaves in pot-pourri and the flowers for trimmings.

Ageratum houstonianum
Ageratum
Blue, white or pink clustered flowerheads that look like shaving brushes. Hang upside-down to air dry. Blue varieties dry best.

Ammobium
Ammobium
Tiny white daisy-like flowers. Hang upside-down and dry in a warm place. Keep pure white color well. Remove untidy leaves. Use in pot-pourris.

Alchemilla mollis
Lady's mantle
Small flowers grow in a yellow-green mass. Air dry upright. Use the leaves in pot-pourri and the flowers in arrangements.

Anaphalis
Anaphalis or pearl everlasting
Clusters of white flowers form flowerheads which dry well; the attractive foliage is gray. Do not remove the leaves from the stem and hang to air dry or leave to dry upright. Use in pot-pourris.

Anemone
Anemone or windflower
Cup-shaped flowers with petals which open out flat when mature. Dry the fragile flowers in silica gel to trim pot-pourris.

Angelica archangelica
Angelica
Chop up the roots in their first fall before they become woody and dry to use as a fixative in pot-pourris. Pick the leaves to air dry before flowering; break up to add greenery and fragrance to pot-pourris.

Anthemis nobilis
Chamomile
Correct name is *Chamaemelum nobile,* but usually available as *Anthemis.* The daisy-like flowers air dry well. Use in sachets.

Aristea
African iris
A pinkish-brown, reed-like growth of small, bell-shaped flowers. Useful in pot-pourris.

Artemesia abrotanum
Southernwood or lad's love
Grows in a feathery mass of narrow, pointed leaves; dried they retain their green color. Its unpleasant smell deters moths.

Artemesia vulgaris
Mugwort
Tiny gray-green bobbly flowers that grow in spikes. Air dry for flower arrangements and for trimmings in pot-pourris.

Artocarpus heterothyllus
Jack fruit
Grayish-brown spiky ovoids like little hedgehogs. Use in exotic and spicy pot-pourris.

Astrantia major
Masterwort
Star-like greenish-pink flowers on branching stems. Air dry the open flowers; for best results dry in silica. Use in pot-pourris.

Banksia coccinea
Protea
Large flowers that look like an elongated, less compact artichoke. Air dry to trim pot-pourris and for dried arrangements.

Bellis perennis
Daisy
Familiar as a lawn weeds. Small, star-like pretty white flowers with a yellow centers. Dry in desiccant to trim pot-pourris.

Betula pendula
Birch
A graceful tree with beautiful pale bark and catkins. The leaves are oval and mid-green; glycerine to preserve.

Borago officinalis
Borage
A culinary herb; air dry the leaves and small sprays of very blue flowers for pot-pourris.

Boswellia carteri
Frankincense
Gum resin can be used in pot-pourris as a fixative. Oil from the resin has a beautiful fragrance.

Bougainvillea
Bougainvillea
Air dry papery bracts in cerise, magenta, scarlet and deep pink. Brilliant colors and lightweight, very useful base for pot-pourris.

Brachychiton
Brachychiton pods
Large, brown, pea-like seedpods which split to reveal a row of rich golden-yellow seeds. Decorative in pot-pourris.

Brassica sp.
Cressia
Woody stems with sparse leaves carrying soft, deep-yellow tufty flowers. Useful in dried arrangements or to trim pot-pourri.

Brunia laevis
Silver brunia
Tight, silver-gray bobbles grow in clusters on fine, slightly scaly stems. Useful in pot-pourris.

Calamus aromaticus
Calamus
The root has a sweet, aromatic smell; chop to use in pot-pourris.

Calendula officinalis
Marigold
Air dry the bright yellow and orange flowerheads flat for use in pot-pourri. Dry special heads for trimming in silica.

Camellia japonica
Camellia
Bowl-shaped flowers are white, pink or red; dry in silica. The leathery leaves are a glossy dark green and glycerine well, eventually turning shiny brown. Use in pot-pourris or arrangements.

Capsicum
Peppercorns
Small pink berries along a fragile stem air dry well. A decorative addition to pot-pourris and other dried arrangements.

Cassia
Senna
A useful little seedpod, light in weight and soaks up perfume well. Greenish-brown in color. A useful non-floral ingredient for pot-pourris and arrangements.

Cedrus libani
Cedar
The cedar of Lebanon has light, warm-brown, rose-like cones known as "cedar roses" that are flat and flowerlike and look good on wreaths. Also useful in pot-pourris and arrangements.

Celosia argentea cristata
Cock's comb
Crested flowerheads in pink, red, orange or yellow with the look and texture of crumpled velvet. Hang upside-down to air dry. Use pieces in pot-pourri and whole in dried arrangements.

Centaurea cyanus
Cornflower
A slender stem with gray-green leaves and branched sprays of blue, white, pink, red or purple flowers. Cut the stems short and hang upside-down to air dry in a really warm place for pot-pourri.

Cheiranthus cheiri
Wallflower
The flowers are shaped rather like a celtic cross; they come in white, yellow, orange, scarlet, crimson and purple. Dry in silica for trimmings only in pot-pourri.

Chrysanthemum
Chrysanthemum
The large flowerheads are too sappy to dry well. Dry the small, pom-pom heads in silica as pot-pourri trimmings.

Cinnamon zeylanicum
Cinnamon
The quills are the dried inner bark of the shoots. Use broken as pot-pourri ingredients and whole on wreaths and larger-scale floral decorations.

Citrus bergemia
Bergamot
One of the less well-known citrus plants. The peel yields a valuable essential oil. It has the scent of Earl Grey tea.

Clematis
Clematis
Petal-like sepals form a hanging cup or bell. Choose large flower-heads and dry in silica to trim pot-pourris or in arrangements.

Coco nucifera
Coco flower
Flat, anemone-like flowers with a hard, woody texture. Naturally coconut-colored but often dyed. Both flowers and petals are excellent in pot-pourris.

Commiphora myrrha
Myrrh gum
The resin exudes as a gum which dries and is scrapped off. Has a musty, spicy scent. A fixative (and oil) for use in pot-pourri.

Convallaria majalis
Lily-of-the-valley
Delicate arching stems carry five to eight tiny white waxy flowers that are bell-shaped and sweet-scented. For best results dry stems in silica gel crystals. The natural oil is rare; use synthetic.

Coriandrum sativum
Coriander
Use the dried seeds as a carrier materials for spicy pot-pourris.

Corylus avellana
Hazel
Nut-bearing trees and shrubs, the cob nuts are decorative and the twigs useful in pot-pourris.

Cupressus macropcarpa
Cypress
The grayish-beige, heavy cones have a texture like open scales. Goes well with pinks in pot-pourris and arrangements.

Cycas sp.
Palm rings or rams' heads
Enchanting, large seedpods shaped like rams' horns. An excellent trimming for exotic pot-pourris. Use also on swags.

Cymbopogon citratus
Lemon grass
Long, slender bright-green leaves have a lemon flavouring. Use the chopped air-dried leaves in pot-pourris. A strong lemony oil.

Cynara scolymus
Globe artichoke
Air dry the attractive vegetable before it has sprouted its purple flower like a shaving brush. The large silvery leaves are lovely in arrangements and pot-pourris.

Daucus carota
Queen Anne's lace
The wild carrot has feathery leaves and delicate white umbels. Hang to air dry (or water dry) when first in flower before going to seed for pot-pourris and arrangements.

Delphinium
Delphinium
Tall spikes of blue, white, pink, purple and mauve flowers. Hang spikes separately to air dry. Hang *D. consolida* or larkspur in bunches of five or six spikes. Strip flowers off when dry for a good pot-pourri base. For trimmings dry in silica. White doesn't dry well; blue dries best.

Dianthus caryophyllus
Carnation
Wire the heads before drying in silica as they shrivel if air dried. Gray-green buds dry well for use in pot-pourris.

Dipteryx odorata
Tonquin bean
Fragrant, wrinkled black beans are pretty whole in pot-pourris. Use crushed or powdered as carrier for oils. Strongly fixative.

Echinops ritro
Globe thistle
Globular steely-blue flowers with dense spikes and deep gray-green leaves. Stand or hang to dry. Use to trim pot-pourris or in arrangements.

Eleagnus ebbingei
Eleagnus
One side of leaf is shiny, under-side is velvety. Glycerines very well. Most go brown but this variety turns a lovely gold. Use in arrangements.

Elletaria cardamomum
Cardamom
Use whole seeds in pot-pourris for fragrance. The husks (with black seeds removed) are a good carrier for oils in pot-pourris.

Eryngium
Eryngium or sea holly
Teasel-like heads with a silvery or purple-blue metallic sheen. Once the flowerheads are fully developed and begin to turn blue, hang or stand to air dry. Use whole in arrangements.

Eucalyptus
Eucalyptus
There are hundreds of types of trees and shrubs. *E. gunnii*, with blue-green to silver-white round leaves. The glycerined leaves stay gray-green. Air dried they turn anything from pearly gray to brown and purple-brown. Use in pot-pourris and arrangements.

Eucalyptus arachnoida
Spider gum
Spiky greenish-brown gums on branches with a very hard, woody texture. Interesting top dressing for pot-pourris.

Eucalyptus tetragona
Gum sprays
Available fresh as grayish-blue gum nuts on fine branches with a white, almost frosted "powdery" look. Use to top dress pot-pourris and in arrangements.

Eugenia aromatica
Clove
The undeveloped flower buds of the tree have a strong, sweet, spicy fragrance. Use ground, or whole as carrier material in pot-pourri. Also a valuable oil.

Evernia purpuracea
Oakmoss
An attractive seaweedy-like silvery gray lichen that grows on tree trunks, especially the oak tree. An excellent fixative. Use in pot-pourris and arrangements.

Fagus sylvatica
Beech
Pointed leaves with a wavy edge. The young leaves are bright green, maturing to darker green and turning yellow and red in fall. Glycerine or air dry for arrangements. Use mast or seedpods in pot-pourri.

Ferula galbaniflua
Galbanum
The whole plant abounds with a milky juice which hardens to form "tears" of gum resin. A powerful fixative.

Filipendula ulmaria
Meadowsweet
The small leaves are serrated. There are branching, flattened heads of creamy-white fragrant flowers. Hang to air dry. Use in pot-pourris or arrangements.

Fructus ceratoniae
Locust or carob bean
Large, shiny brown bean pods. Rub with oil for fragrance to give contrast and texture to trim a pot-pourri. Also good in winter swags and wreaths.

Galium odoratum
Sweet woodruff
Tiny, white clustered. Pointed leaves grow in circles around a flat-sided stem. The leaves air dry and smell of sweet hay. Use in scented sachets.

Gentiana
Gentian
Trumpet-shaped flowers, usually vivid blue. Preserve the flowers in silica gel to trim pot-pourris.

Gingko biloba
Ginko or maidenhair tree
Press the bright green leaves which turn cinnamon brown, or use them when golden in fall in pot-pourris.

Gomphocarpus physocarpus
Gas plant
Also known as *Asclepias physocarpa*. After flowering, air dry large, puffed green seedpods with soft bristles, like gooseberries. Use to trim pot-pourris.

Gomphrena globosa
Globa amaranth
Rounded flowerheads in orange, yellow, purple, pink or white. Hang upside-down to air dry when open. Use in pot-pourris.

Gypsophila
Gypsophila or baby's breath
Tiny, star-like flowers on delicate stems. Air dry quickly if hung upside-down. Can also water dry. Separate the bunches so they do not tangle. Or glycerine to maintain flexible stems. Use to top dress pot-pourris.

Hedera helix
Ivy
Climbing evergreen with glossy dark green or variegated leaves. Grows in decorative trails. Air dry for use in pot-pourris. Glycerine to preserve: either in usual way or lay trails in shallow bath of solution. Turns olive green and sometimes brown.

Helianthus annuus
Sunflower
Tall, daisy-like flowers with large flowerheads. Use the individual yellow petals in pot-pourris. The miniature varieties air dry; large heads are difficult to dry.

Helichrysum bracteatum
Straw flower or everlasting
Rounded flowerheads with small, dense petals, in many colors. Hang bunches upside-down to air dry just before the flowers are fully open. Use in pot-pourris or arrangements.

Heliotropium
Heliotrope or cherry pie
Intensely fragrant, forget-me-not-like small flowers in many shades from dark violet, through lavender to white. Hang to air dry and use in pot-pourris.

Helleborus orientalis
Hellebore or lenten rose
Saucer-shaped flowers in various shades, including white, pink, crimson and purple. The green and purple large-headed variety are best for drying. Dry in sand as a lovely top dressing for pot-pourris or to decorate a ring.

Hibiscus
Hibiscus
When bought commercially, the dried flowers are crumpled and dark red and act as an effective carrier material, for example used in exotic pot-pourris. The pods are much less expensive than the flowers, these air dry flat and can be rubbed with oil to add fragrance to a mix.

Hyacinthus orientalis
Hyacinth
These bulbs bloom as compact spikes of bell-shaped flowers. Available in a several colors, in particular white, pink and blue. They have a delicious sweet scent. Air dry or silica dry the florets for use in pot-pourris.

Hydrangea macrophylla
Hydrangea
Flowering shrubs that produce globes of dense petals in white, pink, purple and blue. They dry well: make sure that the flowers are mature before attempting to dry. Hang to air dry or water dry. Use whole in arrangements, or in sprigs in pot-pourris.

Illicium verum
Star anise
The fruit of this tree ripens to produce an eight-pointed dark-brown star. The outer casing splits to reveal shiny brown seeds which are good carrier materials. Use in spice rings and decorations.

Iris
Iris
Two types: bulbs and rhizomes. The flowers are made up of three layers of a trio of petals. Come in many shades – white, blue, purple and yellow. Silica dry the flowers. Orris comes from the roots of *I germanica* 'Florentina'.

Jasminum officinalis
Jasmine
Common white jasmine has lots of small, pure white flowers. Air dry leaves and small sprays flat for pot-pourris. Dry whole sprays in silica for pot-pourri trimmings.

Juniperus communis
Juniper
Grows upright with very dense, narrow leaves. The fruits are green, then black before drying. The berries are good carrier materials, adding fragrance and interest to pot-pourris.

Kerria japonica 'Pleniflora'
Bachelor's buttons
A hardy bush with slender branches bearing orange-yellow flowers and bright-green toothed leaves. When the flowers are fully open hang upside-down in small bunches to air dry; for pot-pourri trimmings dry in silica.

Larix decidua
Larch
A tree shaped like a Christmas tree. The cones grow close along the stems and are light-brown through to grayish-brown, sometimes carrying lichen. Pretty in pot-pourri and arrangements.

Laurus nobilis
Bay
Air dry the dark-green, glossy leaves flat, in sprays or singly. Use sprays in arrangements and single leaves in pot-pourri.

Lavandula
Lavender
One of the world's most useful scents comes from these hardy evergreen shrubs; the oil is produced from the tops and stalks. Hang bunches to air dry before the buds open. Use to fill sachets and as a carrier in pot-pourri.

Lignum rhodium
Rosewood
South American wood distilled for oil with a sweet, woody smell.

Lilium
Lily
The typical lily has six petals, often with prominent stamens. Available in a huge range of colors, except blue. Some have long trumpets, others have curved back petals, they are often fragrant and always beautiful. Dry the heads in silica gel for use in arrangements.

Lippia citriodora
Lemon or sweet verbena
Also known as *Aloysia triphylla.* Dried flat, the long, narrow light- to mid-green leaves are useful in lemon and herby pot-pourri.

Liquidambar orientalis
Storax
A gum resin with a vanilla-like scent used in old pot-pourri. Generally obtainable in liquid form today. A good fixative. Storax is also called styrax.

Lunaria annua
Honesty
Requires minimal drying. Remove the outer pods by rubbing gently between thumb and forefinger to reveal the silvery inner pods which are dry and papery, like "pennies" Use in arrangements and pot-pourri.

Magnolia
Magnolia
Beautiful flowering trees or shrubs with large, spectacular star-shaped scented flowers in white, cream and shades of pink. The thick green leaves can be very large. Dry the flowers in silica gel and the leaves in glycerine to trim pot-pourri or for impact in dried arrangements.

Mahonia japonica
Mahonia
Yellow globular flowers on a drooping stem with blue-black berries. Glycerine the dark, glossy leaves for arrangements.

Malva
Mallow
Open funnel-shaped flowers with papery petals. Air dry the heads flat as a good purple pot-pourri ingredient. Silica dry large species for a top dressing.

Matthiola incana
Stock
These scented flowers grow in massed spikes and come in pastel shades and stronger colors. Air dry quickly in a warm place when in full flower. Use the flowers only in pot-pourri or dry as spikes for arrangements.

Melissa officinalis
Lemon balm
A well-loved garden herb also known as "cottager's tea". The dried leaves are lemon-scented and retain their fragrance well. The mid-green, variegated or yellow 'All Gold' leaves are suitable for use in pot-pourri. Air dry flat or hang in bunches.

Mentha
Mint
M. spicata, the common mint or spearmint has tiny pale purple flowers and leafy spikes. Hang bunches to air dry dark-green or variegated leaves for pot-pourri.

Molucella laevis
Bells of Ireland
Tall, fresh green spikes with small, white flowers each surrounded by a large, shell-like pale green calyx. Hang or stand the spikes to air dry. Or glycerine them but note that with this drying method the stems will eventually turn beige, especially if they are exposed to light.

Myristica fragrans
Nutmeg or mace
Nutmeg is a dried seed kernel. The dried outer shell of the nut produces yellowish mace which is more fragrant (and also more costly) than nutmeg. Use whole nutmegs for decoration in pot-pourri, on wreaths etc.

Myroxylon balsamum
Balsam of Peru
Every part of the plant is aromatic and the flowers can be smelt from 100yds distance. It has a thick, honey-like resin with a vanilla-like scent. An excellent fixative.

Myrtus
Myrtle
Useful for its glossy, quite dark green leaves. Air dry the leaves for use in pot-pourri, or you can glycerine them for perfection for use on larger-scale decorations and dried arrangements.

Narcissus
Daffodil
The characteristic trumpet is surrounded by petals that comes in almost every shade between white and orange; some are two-tone. Cut stems short to air dry the flowers flat for pot-pourri. Silica dry good specimens to use as a decorative top dressing.

Nelumbo
Lotus
If available, the rich pink flowers and buds can be silica dried. Air dry the huge bright green leaves and break up for pot-pourris (the whole leaf would line a bowl). Decorative seedheads with a flat, round head full of holes, each containing a large seed. There are two types: the large brownish-gray lotus and the bluish-gray "mini" lotus.

Nicandra physaloides
Shoo fly
Bell-shaped violet flowers and white fruits hide inside bright green and purple calyces. Remove the leaves and hang the mature seedpods like shiny green lanterns to air dry. Use in pot-pourri and arrangements.

Nigella damascena
Love-in-a-mist
Very finely cut foliage and blue, white or pink flowers. The seedpods have purple and green stripes; allow to mature before air drying or they shrivel. Hang the double varieties in bunches to air dry. Use in pot-pourri and dried arrangements.

Nummern gossypium
Cotton husk pods
A by-product of cotton plants, the little star-shaped beige husks are useful in pot-pourri and stuck on wreaths etc.

Nux vomica
Bell cups
Spherical, creamy-beige cups which range between golf-ball and tennis-ball size. Hard and woody, they provide useful pot-pourri trimmings.

Ocimum basilicum
Basil
Oval-shaped, aromatic leaves with a strong, clove-like flavour. Usually mid-green, but purple-leaved varieties are available. Air dry flat for use in pot-pourri.

Omorica
Omorica

Solid, pinkish-brown cones which are long and narrow. Rub with oil (which they absorb well) to give an interesting accent in pot-pourris and arrangements.

Origanum vulgare
Marjoram

Hang up bunches of small, mid-green, rounded leaves to air dry. The 'Aureum' variety has golden-yellow leaves when young. Use in pot-pourris and sachets.

Oroxylum indicum
Angels' wings

Purplish-brown winged seed-heads like little "windmills". They are light, decorative and absorb fragrance when rubbed with oil. Use in pot-pourris.

Paeonia
Peony

The bowl-shaped flowers open out flat when mature. Available in many colors and varieties. Hang stems to air dry and use petals as a base material in pot-pourris. Dry the whole heads in silica gel for trimming and to give impact on wreaths etc. The tree *P. delavayii* produces beautiful star-shaped seedheads and *P. Lutea* has twin seedpods; pick when the pods have split open.

Papver
Poppy

The flowers generally have four broad overlapping petals to form a cup or bowl shape. Air dry whole heads of double varieties for pot-pourri ingredients and trimmings. Or silica dry. The seedheads are very decorative in all sorts of arrangements.

Pavetta indica
Gum nuts or papri cups

Little grayish-brown woody seedheads which look like clay pipes without their stems. Excellent pot-pourri ingredients and can be used on wreaths etc

Pelargonium
Geranium

The air-dried leaves are mid-green and variegated. Use in pot-pourris or press for a top dressing. Provides a useful oil.

Philadelphus
Double mock orange

The white cup-shaped flowers have a strong fragrance that is reminiscent of orange blossom. Air dry the fresh green leaves flat while they are still young. Dry flower sprays likewise, but preserve sprays in silica gel for top dressing pot-pourris.

Physalis alkekengii
Chinese lantern

After the small, white flowers have appeared, bright red calyces follow which enclose an edible orange berry; these most decorative orange papery fruits provide useful decoration for arrangements. Hang upside-down to air dry the seedpods.

Pimento dioica
Allspice

A composite spice fragrance and staple ingredient of traditional pot-pourris, crushed, powdered or whole. Use whole as a carrier material in pot-pourri mixes.

Pinus
Pine

Coniferous trees characterized by needle-like leaves changing from light to dark green as they mature. Most useful for woody cones in all shades of gray and brown and in many forms; some are banana-shaped and some like miniature pineapples. Suitable for use in winter arrangements and pot-pourris.

Pithecellobium dulce
Curly pods

Light pinkish-brown split seed-pods with naturally curly forms. Strong and light – an excellent base material for pot-pourris. Often found in dyed colors.

Pogostemon patchouli
Patchouli

It is very difficult to obtain the leaf of this plant for it is distilled in India for its wonderful oil.

Polianthes tuberosa
Tuberose

Heavily scented flowers in pure white on erect spikes; each flower has six open petals that grow from a funnel-shaped tube. Because this is a fleshy flower it needs to be air dried for some time for use in pot-pourri.

Polyanthus
Polyanthus

Primrose-like flowers with short stems, they derive from *Primula vulgaris*. They are found in many colors and are widely available as commercially grown flowers, usually potted. For best results dry the flowers in silica gel. They provide a decorative trimming for pot-pourris, wreaths etc.

Polygonum bistorta
Snakeweed

The variety 'Superbum' has spikes of closely set pink flowers and large oval-shaped light green leaves. Hang upside-down to air dry for use in pot-pourris.

Polypodium vulgare
Polybody fern

A commonly seen fern in Britain, it can spread over large areas. The mid-green fronds droop elegantly. Do not pick while the spores are active, as they are carcinogenic; wait until the spores are inactive. As with all ferns, they are most successfully preserved by pressing between sheets of paper. Use whole for decoration, or broken up as a pot-pourri ingredient.

Polyporous perrenis
Golden mushroom

Umbrella-shaped mushrooms in every shade of brown, from pale to almost black. Useful as decorative additions to pot-pourris.

Populus candicans
Balm of Gilead

A fragrant poplar with pale green leaves which emit a strong balsamic smell. The buds are useful in pot-pourris. True balm of Gilead, mentioned in the Bible, is *Commiphora opobalsamum* which is extremely expensive.

Preigo
Pregio "nails"

Large and black, these have the appearance of iron nails, giving dark contrast in pot-pourris.

Primula vulgaris
Primrose

Familiar growing in wild spaces, these flowers have corrugated mid-green leaves and clusters of low-growing pale yellow blooms with darker yellow centers. For best results preserve the flowers in silica gel crystals. Do not pick the leaves or the plant will be destroyed. Use in pot-pourris.

Prunus laurocerasus
Laurel

A shrub with pointed, leathery leaves. It bears small dark fruits and white flowers. The Portugal laurel (*P. lausitanica*) has glossy dark green leaves with red stalks and cream, scented flowers; some have white-variegated leaves. Like most leaves, for best results preserve in glycerine. Use whole in arrangements or broken up in pot-pourris.

Pseudoacacia semprevirens
Flora de Madeira

Grayish-brown, tulip-like seed-pods with an attractive architectural quality that makes them useful as pot-pourri trimmings and on swags and garlands

Pterocarpus macrocarpus
Pradu flowers

Flat, large brown-papery seed-heads with a grayish tinge. Lightweight and strong, they make excellent pot-pourri base ingredients or trimmings.

Quercus
Oak
A long-living tree; the leaves are deeply lobed and can assume rich fall colors. The fruits are the well-known acorns or nuts held in a cup-like husk; these air dry naturally and are useful for decoration. Glycerine the leaves while still young – they look lovely on wreaths.

Ranunculaceae asiaticus
Ranunculus
Lovely, fat double balls of petals in many shades with a papery texture. Hang upside-down to air dry or dry to perfection in silica.

Reseda
Mignonette
This upright plant has a tuft of orange-yellow stamens and small yellow-white flowers. It is valued for its fragrance. Air dry for fragrant pot-pourri ingredient.

Rosa
Rose
There are enormous numbers of roses, including old roses, hybrid teas, floribunda, shrub, climbers and miniatures. The staple ingredient of moist pot-pourri, the rose remains as important today. Before the flowers are fully open hang stems in small bunches to air dry in a warm place or dry heads or sprays in silica. Reserve loose petals for pot-pourri.

Rosmarinus officinalis
Rosemary
The strongly aromatic leaves are narrow and mid to dark green with a white underside; the shoots are distilled to make oil. Hang or stand sprays of foliage to air dry for use in pot-pourri.

Ruta graveolens
Rue
An old strewing herb. The sap can cause blisters to the skin. The plant has clusters of yellow flowers and blue-green leaves. Air dry for use in sachets.

Salix
Willow
There are all sorts of willows, their decorative catkins and furry pussy willow twigs are useful in pot-pourris and arrangements.

Salvia officinalis
Sage
An aromatic evergreen bush with soft, hairy almost velvety gray-green leaves and tiny flowers. Use in herb arrangements and to top dress pot-pourri.

Salvia sclarea
Clary
The leaves are large, hairy and pungently aromatic; the flowers are tubular and blue-white and grow on tall stems. Hang to air dry for use in pot-pourris.

Santalum album
Sandalwood
Every part of the wood is used: the sawdust makes sachets and the raspings are a good carrier and fixative in dry pot-pourri. The essential oil is wonderful.

Sorbus aucuparia
Rowan or mountain ash
Mid green leaves with a gray underside, turning yellow in fall. The flowers are followed by bunches of orange-red berries. Hang to air dry. Use in pot-pourris and arrangements.

Spiraea
Spiraea
Attractive flowering shrubs with small, star-like flowers that grow alongside pale-green leaves on slender, arching branches. For best results dry in desiccant. Use sprigs to trim pot-pourri.

Stachys lanata
Lamb's ears
Also known as lamb's tongue. A low-growing plant with small purple flowers and oval-shaped leaves covered with dense white hairs to give a woolly texture. Air dry for use in pot-pourris.

Styrax benzoin
Gum benzoin
A strongly fixative gum that is collected from wounded tree bark; the hardened resin "almonds" are scrapped off. Used in dry form in pot-pourris and incenses. A valuable oil much used in spicy blends.

Syringa vulgaris
Lilac
Shrubs and small trees carrying fragrant, small, dense flowers, in lilac, pink or white. Hang upside-down to air dry or dry in desiccant for use in pot-pourris.

Tagetes erecta
African marigold
Daisy-like yellow flowers with deep cut, dark shiny leaves that are strongly scented. Hang to air dry for use in pot-pourris; they retain color well. Dry in silica or sand as trimmings.

Tanacetum
Tansy
Dense clusters of yellow flowers with lacy leaves. Leave sprays on the stem to air dry. A moth herb which has rather an unpleasant smell; do not use in pot-pourris, but use in sachets.

Thymus citriodorus
Lemon thyme
This species has broader leaves than *T. vulgaris*. When crushed, the leaves give off a strong, lemon scent. Use in pot-pourris.

Thymus vulgaris
Thyme
The dark, very small narrow leaves are aromatic and carry clusters of small, mauve flowers. Air dry for herby pot-pourris.

Trameles betulius
Sponge mushroom
A beautiful Indian fungus that comes in all shades of cream and beige. When dried it has the appearance of carved wood. Use in pot-pourris and arrangements.

Tulipa
Tulip
A goblet-shaped flower with six petals standing on an erect stem. The petals come in a huge range of colors: rounded, pointed, double and with frilled edges. Large parrot tulips have striped petals. Air dry heads and petals for pot-pourri. Dry in silica for perfect flowerheads to top dress.

Vetiveria zizannoides
Vetiver
The thin, wiry roots of this grass emit the sharp, rooty scent of vetiver; it is a powerful fixative.

Viola odorata
Violet
The highly scented flowers come in shades of purple or white with heart-shaped leaves. Dry large varieties in silica gel and press the leaves for use in pot-pourris.

Viola tricolor
Pansy
Available in cream and yellow through to dark blue and purple-black, or sometimes bicolored. They retain their color well when dried in silica gel. Make a lovely top dressing for pot-pourri and useful on wreaths etc.

Zea mays
Corn cob
Miniature varieties are most useful in pot-pourris and wreaths. Large types come in yellow and dark red; miniatures in yellow, gold, red and "blue".

Zingiber officinale
Ginger
Strong-smelling whole or sliced, dried ginger root can be used in pot-pourris in small quantities.

Zinnia
Zinnia
Cheerful, colorful daisy-like flowers with dense petals. Hang upside-down in bunches to air dry, or silica dry specimens for top dressing pot-pourris.

LIST OF SUPPLIERS

IN THE UK

Angela Flanders
Highfield House
Lower Blandford Road
Shaftesbury
Dorset SP7 8NR
*Mail order and general information.
Hand-made pot-pourris and room
fragrancing products. Plus all sorts
of pot-pourri materials and essential
oils, dried plants, gums and
balsams, spices and fixatives. Full
range of oils ready blended to make
the recipes in this book.*

Caroline Alexander
The Hop Shop
Castle Farm
Shoreham
Kent TN14 7UB
*Retail. Growers and driers of
English flowers. Offering an
extensive range of fine-quality dried
flowers and hops in season.*

Baldwin's
171-173 Walworth Road
London SE17 1RW
*Medical herbalists. Retail and mail
order. Offering an extensive range
of pot-pourri materials, essential
oils, fixatives, dried plants, gums,
balsams and spices.*

Maggie Berry and Pippa Palmers
Manor Flowers of Brenley
The Old Granary
Brenley Farm
Boughton-under-Blean
Faversham
Kent ME13 9LY
*Retail. Growers and suppliers of
ready-dried English garden flowers,
with some more unusual varieties
also available.*

Elizabeth Bullivant
Stourton House Flower Garden
Stourton
Near Warminster
Wiltshire BA12 6QF
*Dried English garden flowers,
unusual glycerined leaves,
specialist plants.*

Candle Makers Supplies
28 Blythe Road
Hammersmith
London W14 OHA
*Candle-making equipment. Mail
order for paraffin, beeswax, wicks,
moulds, dyes etc.*

Culpeper Shops
Head office
21 Bruton Street
London W1X 7DA
*Retail. Stock a wide range of
essential oils at sensible prices, plus
many herbs and pot-pourri
fixatives. Branch shops are located
nationwide.*

Carl Grover
C. M.Grover Ltd
Stands N5 and N6
New Covent Garden Market
Nine Elms Lane
London SW8
*The Grover family have a market
stall at Columbia Road, London E2
on Sunday mornings.*

Hambledon Herbs
Court Farm
Milverton
Somerset TA4 1NF
*Wholesale. Offer a wide range of
organic flowers and herbs for pot-
pourr making. Minimum quantity
half kg of each variety.*

Brian Lee
Tudorose Dried Flowers
15 Carronade Place
Broadwaters
West Thamesmead
London SE28 0EE
*Wholesale van service. Good range
of English and Dutch dried flowers.
Freeze-dried flowers, fruit and
vegetables, exotic pods etc.
Minimum order £100.*

New Covent Garden Market
Nine Elms Lane
London SW8
*Wholesale market with sundries
merchants permanently based,eg
Pollards, Coquerelles and Donovans.*

Organics
The Old Stables
98 Ravenscroft Street
London E2 7QA
*Retail. Stocks exotics: pods, roots,
leaves and mosses. Flower arranging
materials, willow rings and baskets.*

Richard Witherden
Peerless Importing Company
Dee Mill
Llangollen LL20 8SD
*Wholesale. Information on stockists.
Range of dried flowers and exotics:
pods, cones, barks and mosses.*

IN THE USA

Caswell Massey
Catalogue Division
111 Eighth Avenue
New York
NY 10011
*Wide range of oils, dried plant
materials, fixatives, herbs, gums
and spices.*

Indiana Botanic Gardnes
PO Box 5 HA
Hammon
IN 46325
*Extensive list of essential oils and
other materials.*

Penn Herb Co.
Dept HA
603 N 2nd Street
Philadelphia
PA 19123
Oils and other pot-pourri materials.

San Francisco Herb Company
250 14th Street
San Francisco
CA 94103
*Wide range of oils and other pot-
pourri making materials.*

Tom Thumb Workshops
Box 332
Chincoteague
VA 23336
*Extensive list of essential oils and
dried materials, exotic pods and
dried flowers.*

IN CANADA

Wild Thyme Herb Company
Box 20212
Calgary Place Postal Outlet
T2P 4J3
*Organic herbs, pot-pourri materials
and seminars on herbs.*

Note that most health shops and
some druggists now stock a range
of essential oils and herbs and some
may be able to order fixatives such
as orris and gum benzoin on
demand.

BIBLIOGRAPHY

Bullivant, Elizabeth, *Dried Fresh Flowers*, Pelham Books, 1989

Culpeper, Nicholas, *The Complete Herbal*, first published 1653

Davis, Patricia, *Subtle Aromatherapy*, C.W. Daniel Co Ltd, 1991

Foster, Maureen, *The Flower Arranger's Encyclopedia of Preserving and Drying*, Blandford Press, 1988

Genders, Roy, *Perfume through the Ages*, New York, 1972; *Scented Flora of the World*, London, 1977

Gerard, John, *The Historie of Plants*, 1597

Grieve, Mrs M, FRHS, *A Modern Herbal*, first published by Jonathan Cape 1931, revised edition 1973; Tiger Book International 1992

Jekyll, Gertrude, *Home and Garden*

Le Guérer, Annick, *Scent*, Chatto & Windus, London, 1993

Morris, Edwin, T., *Fragrance*, E.T. Morris & Co, Greenwich, Connecticut, New York, 1984

Ohrbach, Barbara Milo, *The Scented Room*, Clarkson N. Potter Inc, New York, 1986

Paolo, Rosvesti, *In Search of Perufmes Lost*, Blow Up Press, Venice, 1980

Piesse, G.W. Septimus, *The Art of Perfumery*, Longman, Brown, Green and Longmans, London, 1855

Platt, Sir Hugh, *Delights for Ladies*, reprinted 1948

Poucher, William, *Perfumes, Cosmetics and Soaps*, Van Nostrand & Co, New York, 1926

Rohde, Eleanor Sinclair, *Rose Recipes*, Routledge, 1939; *The Old English Herbals*, *The Scented Garden*, Medici Society, London

The Toilet of Flora, 1775

Theodore, James, *The Pot Pourri Gardener*, Macmillan Publishing Co, New York

Thompson, C.J.S., *The Mystery and Lure of Perfumes*, Bodley Head, London, 1927

Tisserand, Robert, *Aromatherapy for Everyone*, Arkana, 1990; *The Art of Aromatherapy*, C.W. Daniel Co Ltd, 1977

Valnet, Dr Jean, *The Practise of Aromatherapy*, C.W. Daniel Co Ltd, 1980

Worwood, Valerie Ann, *The Fragrant Pharmacy*, Macmillan London Ltd, 1990

HAZARDOUS ESSENTIAL OILS

Essential oils are very strong and must be used with care. Certain oils should not be used under the following conditions:

Pregnancy
Basil, birch, cedarwood, clary sage, cypress, fennel, hyssop, jasmine, juniper, marjoram, myrrh, peppermint, rose otto, rosemary and thyme.

Epilepsy
Fennel (sweet), hyssop, rosemary and sage.

Sensitive skin
Basil, fennel, lemon, lemongrass, lemon verbena, melissa, peppermint and sage, thyme or tea tree. Do not use cinnamon oil on the skin at all.

High blood pressure
Hyssop, rosemary, sage and thyme.

Sunshine
Do not use the following oils before exposure to strong sunlight: bergamot, cumin, grapefruit, lemon, lemongrass, melissa, mandarin, lime, orange, verbena or any other citrus fruit.

The following oils, while safe to use in aromatic recipes are not recommended for use on the skin or in other therapeutic situations: calamus, cinnamon, clove (bud and leaf), hyssop and pine.

Never take essential oils internally. Do not use oils in any therapeutic situation without qualified prescription.

INDEX

142

ACKNOWLEDGMENTS

This book would not have been possible without the help and encouragement of a great many people, not only during the time that it has taken to produce, but long before that. It is the culmination of my ten years at Columbia Road and I would like to take this opportunity of thanking all those who have helped me along the way, together with the people of Bethnal Green who took me and my little shop to their hearts and supported and encouraged me in the early days. Thanks to all my customers over the years, so many of whom became friends, likewise the shopkeepers and Sunday flower market traders in Columbia Road, especially Butch and Kip who began it all by finding me the shop, and Carl Grover for supplying me with so many wonderful flowers. Tim and Jacqueline Woolgar of Hybrid Gallery, and Simon and Sue Rees at No 94, for all the faxes and for being such good neighbours. The many people who contributed in various capacities to the cheerful and efficient running of the shop are too numerous to mention individually, but I would especially like to thank Carl Forrest for five years' help in the shop and for his unfailing charm to the customers. And also Lizzi Freeman, who has always been a rich source of inspiration and encouragement.

I have spent much of the last 18 months commuting between Dorset and London, an exercise which would have been quite impossible without the help of Jim Adams and Bob Hopkins of Shaftesbury; my grateful thanks to them for keeping things going at Highfield during my absences.

I have particularly valued the loyal support and interest shown by all my suppliers over the years. Special thanks are due to: Brian Lee of Tudorose Dried Flowers, who supported and encouraged me right from the start, and gave me much wise advice. Rosemary Massouras and David Cressey Hall of the Appledore Co. Ltd, Nottingham, for all the information and help, and the interest that they have always shown in my work. Tim Arnold and Hilary Bosley of Pierce A. Arnold & Son Ltd have been unfailingly helpful and kind, and my thanks are also due to Richard Witherden of Peerless Importing Co. for the exotic ingredients and supplying so many Latin plant names. Jane Pinkster of Church Farm House, Barwick, and Elizabeth Bullivant of Stourton House, Stourton, supplied many of the beautifully grown and dried English garden flowers that we photographed. I should also like to thank Mr Hawkes and Eric Doughty at the Spice Mill for all their courteous help, and John and Luke Whowell for their interest in all my enterprises, and for teaching me so much about fragrance.

I owe a huge debt of gratitude to Judith More and Jacqui Small for finding me at the Country Living Fair and offering me the opportunity to create this book; my grateful thanks to both of them. Thanks to Sophie Pearse, my guiding light, whose patience, calm and understanding under pressure were phenomenal; thanks Sophie, I couldn't have done it without you. And to Sarah Widdicombe for her editorial input. It was an inspiration and a delight to work with Simon Wheeler, whose magical photographs are such an important part of this book and I would like to thank him for his wizardry in photographing all the weird and wonderful things with which I presented him. Penny Stock put in an enormous amount of meticulous work on the visual side and the result says much for her talents. Thanks also to Polly Wreford who photographed the step-by-step projects, and was a joy to work with.

Writing a book is, of necessity, a single-minded, almost obsessive business, and words cannot express my gratitude to my family and friends, who not only fed and nurtured me, but supported and encouraged me at every stage – without their belief in me it would have been a much less enjoyable task.

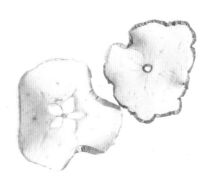